ASEXUAL EROTICS

ABNORMATIVITIES: QUEER/GENDER/EMBODIMENT
Scott Herring, Series Editor

# ASEXUAL EROTICS

## INTIMATE READINGS OF COMPULSORY SEXUALITY

### ELA PRZYBYLO

THE OHIO STATE UNIVERSITY PRESS

COLUMBUS

Library of Congress Cataloging-in-Publication Data
Names: Przybylo, Ela, 1985– author.
Title: Asexual erotics : intimate readings of compulsory sexuality / Ela Przybylo.
Other titles: Abnormativities: queer/gender/embodiment.
Description: Columbus : The Ohio State University Press, [2019] | Series: Abnormativities: queer/gender/embodiment | Includes bibliographical references and index.
Identifiers: LCCN 2019009059 | ISBN 9780814214046 (cloth ; alk. paper) | ISBN 0814214045 (cloth ; alk. paper)
Subjects: LCSH: Asexuality (Sexual orientation) | Sex. | Sexual attraction. | Queer theory. | Feminist theory.
Classification: LCC HQ23 .P78 2019 | DDC 306.7—dc23
LC record available at https://lccn.loc.gov/2019009059

Cover design by Susan Zucker
Text design by Juliet Williamson
Type set in Adobe Minion Pro

# CONTENTS

# ILLUSTRATIONS

# ACKNOWLEDGMENTS

POET LEAH LAKSHMI PIEPZNA-SAMARASINHA writes that in life, "you're going to find the people you can sketch the secret inside of the world with [and] if you can't find them you can sketch the secret inside of your world inside yourself."[1] *Asexual Erotics* was created just in this way—navigating intimacy, distance, betweenness, longing, and loneliness across cities, across contexts, and in erotic entanglement with many people. This book is in remembrance of erotic friendships that were cut short, especially those with Andrzej Przybyło and Jadwiga Chabasińska née Wilczyńska, for instilling in me a sense of longing for erotic worlds past and future. My father, Andrzej Przybyło, showed me Polish soft masculinity at its best, even within contexts of displacement and poor working conditions, teaching me to apply love, pride, and beer breaks to everything one does, both big and small. The biggest of thanks to my intelligent, sassy, and fiercely loving mother, Irena Przybyło née Chabasińska, who has always oriented me toward learning in all its many forms and gifted me with feminist determination and life invention in the face of immigration's many adversities. Despite our differences, I am your daughter through and through and you are my deepest love. Thank you also to both my beautiful Polish femme sisters, Aleksandra Przybyło and Ewa Przybyło, who taught me how to live in ways that were expansive by introducing me to poetry, conversation, writing essays, drawing plants, going on bike rides, traveling on a dime, putting on eyeliner, and loving deeply. Thank you to their children, Veronika, Amelia, and Antoni, for reminding me of the spontaneity of erotic joy through collaging, painting, and play. My heart, as always, is with you my very queer nuclear kin: my nieces and nephew, my mother, my sisters—thank you for being my horizon. Thank you also to our family friend, Elwira Sokołowski, who passed away as I was completing this book and who brought warmth, kindness, and healing into our home during traumatic times.

At The Ohio State University Press, I was fortunate to receive support from an incredible editorial team, including my editor Tara Cyphers, series editor Scott Herring, assistant acquisitions editor Becca Bostock, assistant editor Kristina Wheeler, copyeditor Rebecca S. Bender, marketing director Laurie Avery, and Eugene O'Connor, who took interest in my book project as an acquiring editor. A special thank you also to Benjamin Kahan, KJ Cerankowski, and anonymous reviewers for critical engagements, which made *Asexual Erotics* a much stronger book than it would have been otherwise.

I have been very fortunate also to have exceptional instructors and supervisors throughout my career who provided me with space to learn and the tools with which to develop my research on asexuality. In particular, my thanks to Michelle Meagher, Mebbie Bell, Lise Gotell, Jo-Ann Wallace, and Susanne Luhmann in the Women's and Gender Studies Program at the University of Alberta, who taught me theories and methods that stimulated my feminist imagination. Thank you especially to Michelle Meagher for her continued intellectual support and guidance. Thank you also to faculty both in and beyond the Gender, Feminist, and Women's Studies Graduate Program at York University, including Shannon Bell, Sheila Cavanagh, Barbara Crow, and Eva Karpinski. My biggest thanks to Shannon Bell, who believed that asexuality was a "sexy" topic and encouraged my writing with many prezis, lunches, and the occasional trip in her femme jeep. The biggest thank you to my heart-core feminist friends at York University and especially to Sara Rodrigues, Danielle Cooper, Sage Milo, Veronika Novoselova, Leyna Lowe, Hans Rollmann, Amy Verhaeghe, and Preity Kumar, who have all been part of this project and forever are part of my personal archive of asexual erotics. Thank you to Danielle Cooper in particular for recommending that I look at the "Sisterhood Feels Good" poster featured in chapter 1 and for suggesting that I think about the lesbian art histories of the bed in chapter 2.

I was funded by the Michael Smith Foreign Study Supplement to spend a semester at the University of Auckland in 2010 as part of the Gender and Critical Psychology Research Group, and would like to thank Nicola Gavey, Virginia Braun, and Gareth Terry for their hospitality and collaboration during my time there. At Arizona State University I had the privilege of building friendships with many wonderful folk, including Breanne Fahs, Eric Swanson, Tess Doezema, Jenny Dyck Brian, and the members of the Feminist Research on Gender and Sexuality Group. My most deep feminist gratitude to Breanne Fahs in the Women and Gender Studies Program, who offered me feminist mentorship, encouraged me to put together my book proposal, and became my feminist collaborator and movie theater date. I also want to offer a shout-out to all the queer folk of the Cornell School of Theory and Criticism, 2014 for providing me with an unforgettable summer of karaoke, queer angst, and intimacies. Thank you as well to the many other people who have offered me informal mentorship, including Chloë Taylor, Lucas Crawford, and Kelly Fritsch. My gratitude also to my colleagues in the Department of Gender, Sexuality, and Women's Studies at Simon Fraser University for their support of my work and in particular to Coleman Nye, Helen Hok-Sze Leung, and Lara Campbell, and to Kate Hennessy at the School of Interactive Arts and Technology. Thank you also to Roberta Neilson, who has offered me support at SFU and helped me navigate many a bureaucratic form.

This book would have not been possible without the existence of multiple asexual and asexuality studies communities. In particular, thank you to the Ace/Aro Vancouver, BC community for inviting me to events and for trusting me to be part of the community as an organizer, facilitator, and friend. Thank you in particular to Justine Munich, who has been a source of wisdom and a superb co-organizer. Big gratitude as well to everyone involved in organizing and attending the inaugural asexuality studies conference held in Vancouver in April 2019, "Unthinking Sex, Imagining Asexuality: Intersectional and Interdisciplinary Perspectives," and most especially to my co-organizer, KJ Cerankowski. I am also indebted to the Asexuality Studies Research Group at the National Women's Studies Association, including to Kristina Gupta, KJ Cerankowski, Ianna Hawkins Owen, Eunjung Kim, Cynthia Barounis, Regina Wright, M. Milks, Anna Kurowicka, CJ Chasin, Jasmine Stork, Michael Paramo, Bauer, and others for working together to make asexuality matter in feminist and queer contexts. Thank you also to Steve Davies, who has provided me with many excellent ace-relevant content and asexual resonances and to Theresa Kenney, who has been a fantastic co-collaborator in bringing asexuality to the Sexuality Studies Association and to Women's and Gender Studies et Recherches Féministes in Canada. This book has also benefited from my incredible students and most especially those in "Critical Nonsexualities" at SFU in fall 2017 and students in my asexuality studies directed readings, Evelyn Elgie and Kaiya Jacob, who challenged me to think about erotics and asexuality in many ways both surprising and familiar. This book is for you and for all future asexuality studies scholars.

Finally, thank you to my circles of friends, and especially to my queer pals and rock-climbing buddies who have given me opportunities to laugh at myself, to laugh at them, and to keep the machine of my life oiled by encouraging me to seek learning and momentum through my body. My biggest thanks to my many emotional and thinking interlocutors in Toronto, Phoenix, Vancouver, Edmonton, and beyond with whom I am grateful to have shared love and loving of many forms. To all my erotic friendships past and present for helping me keep loneliness at bay. In particular thank you to my dear friends: Sage Milo for listening and feeding my heart and body; Danielle Cooper for always asking difficult and cranky questions and teaching me how to dress to queer parties; and Sara Rodrigues for being my true friend across changing contexts and identities. Further thanks to my fellow femme traveler Veronika Novoselova, writing companion Leyna Lowe, picketing fellow Amy Verhaeghe, dream roommate Marlo Carpenter, as well as to Stevie Ballantyne, Ada Jaarsma, Tess Doezema, Derek Warwick, Ai Yamamoto, Ania Mariet, and Michael Holly for the gift of friendship, food, romance, and intimacy in many forms. I also want to show gratitude to everyone who has worked with me on the peer-reviewed, open access, and intermedia journal *Feral Feminisms* for creating a base from which to explore feminist praxis.

My gratitude goes to Bracha L. Ettinger for allowing me to feature her incredible art, "Notebook," on the cover of *Asexual Erotics*. The piece is a page excerpted from her artist notebook and speaks to me of the complexity of erotics as well as the capacious possibilities of asexuality. Thank you also to the artists and galleries who provided me with permission to reprint the exquisite art in this monograph and whose visual engagements with queerness made it possible for me to remain invested in the possibilities of erotics, including to Kyle Lasky, Vivek Shraya, Donna Gottschalk, and Tammy Rae Carland. Special thanks to Maisha for the wondrous zine, *Taking the Cake: An Illustrated Primer on Asexuality,* that is a must-read for anyone learning about asexuality. Parts of the introduction were first printed as "Asexuality" in *The Global Encyclopedia of Lesbian, Gay, Bisexual, Transgender and Queer History*; thank you to Cengage for permission to reprint these sections here. Portions of the first chapter are forthcoming in the edited Routledge collection *Rethinking Women's and Gender Studies II,* edited by Ann Braithwaite and Catherine Orr.

Thank you to the Ruth Wynn Woodward Endowment for financing my time at SFU and to the Social Sciences and Humanities Research Council for providing the bread and butter of my funding over the last ten years and during my time at SFU and ASU in particular. Without this funding, the writing of this book as well as my pursuit of research on asexuality would be unthinkable. My gratitude as well to the Government of Alberta, IODE Canada, CUPE 3903, The Institute for the Study of Teaching and Learning in the Disciplines at SFU, SFU's University Publications Fund, Office of the Vice-President Academic at SFU, and the Faculty of Arts and Social Sciences at SFU, for providing funding throughout the writing arc of this book.

This book was completed and has benefited from the bounty of unceded Coast Salish Territory, the traditional territories of the Musqueam, Squamish, Tsleil-Waututh and Kwikwetlem First Nations.

# Erotics and Asexuality

*Thinking Asexuality, Unthinking Sex*

IN HIS spoken word piece "A Prude's Manifesto" (2015), poet Cameron Awkward-Rich announces an asexuality rarely heard or articulated. It is voluminous, erotic, and charged with a longing and desire not easily reducible to sex or sexual attraction. He writes, "Here is a list of things I like more than having sex: Reading. Lying flat on my back staring at the ceiling. Peeling back the skin of a grapefruit. . . . Riding my bike away from parties. How the night swallows me like a dragon. The wet heat of one body alone."[1] He continues, "Love is a girl who slept beside me barely touching for two years. Love is whatever kept us fed. And this is how we knew that we belonged to it." And finally he questions the narrative that self-love and fulfillment need to rely on sex and orgasm, since "if orgasm is really what makes the body sacred then the best love I have ever known was sin or sacrilege."

Awkward-Rich's poetic manifesto, spoken with care and attention, with pause and intensity, invites us into an erotic landscape that opens up erotic energies not tethered to sex. On the one hand, "A Prude's Manifesto" directs us to a deep critique of the effects that compulsory sexuality enacts on asexually abundant lives.[2] By compulsory sexuality, I am referring to a term developed within asexuality studies that, drawing on Adrienne Rich's term "compulsory heterosexuality," speaks to the ways in which sexuality is presumed to be natural and normal to the detriment of various forms of asexual and nonsexual lives, relationships, and identities.[3] Awkward-Rich's poem provides a deep

1

critique of compulsory sexuality by directing our attention to how claims of prudery can be used to mark a subject as backwards, repressed, insufficiently eroticized, and lacking. Sex is too often understood, in Awkward-Rich's words, as "holy," the marker of the successful love, relationship, and individuality, and orgasm is understood to make the body "sacred." For Awkward-Rich, sex can be a narrative we are encouraged to adhere to, an imposition of loving, such that "so often, when someone tells me that I should just love myself it sounds more like they would like me to let them love me the way they want to." Through exploring nonsexual forms of self-fulfillment, moments of joy, and relationship-building, Awkward-Rich rewrites this compulsively sexual narrative of loving and puts forward nonsexual ways of being as erotic in their own right. The prude offers here an erotic figure, which is less an identity and more a description of varying erotic modes that include forms of relating not encompassed by existing sexual identity categories. These erotic modes are both profound and mundane; they are in many ways the "ordinary affects" that Kathleen Stewart writes on, "attending to things . . . already somehow present in them in a state of potentiality or resonance."[4] This prudish asexuality is affirmative yet not predictably identificatory, celebratory yet also complex and fluid. Through an elaboration of multiple modes of nonsexual attracting as well as a politicized talking back to structures that frame orgasm and sex as the ultimate goal of personal and interrelational realization, Awkward-Rich's words provide a perfect opening to a book on thinking about the erotics of asexuality, and the asexuality of erotics.

*Asexual Erotics: Intimate Readings of Compulsory Sexuality* strives to explore both erotic representations of asexuality as well as to develop asexuality as a series of perspectives from which sexuality can be examined. As such, it takes for granted that asexuality is a "legitimate" sexual identity and orientation—that is, that asexuality offers a unique series of identifications that together constitute a distinct orientatory outlook on relating, intimacy, and sociality. Yet while this book takes for granted that asexuality is "real" (an affordance it is routinely denied) and a valid identificatory position and orientation, it does not adhere to the constraints and parameters of contemporary asexual identification as they take form both in online articulations of asexuality and in media representations. The leading online gathering space of asexual knowledge and community formation, the Asexual Visibility and Education Network (AVEN), succinctly describes "an asexual person [as] a person who does not experience sexual attraction."[5] This definition, while complicated and expanded throughout the website, forums, and online and offline community at large, has, since I began doing research on asexuality nearing on a decade ago, sat uneasily with me for its unnuanced rendition of asexual experiences and dispositions. Is asexuality really reducible to an absence of sexual attraction? What is lost when we hinge asexuality, as well as other sexual orientations, to the mechanism of "attraction"? What is the relationship at play between attracting and relating, attracting and desire, attracting and sex? This book's refusal to be bound solely by identificatory frames is strongly motivated by my feeling that while in many ways I tend toward asexuality, the definition as it is pivoted by AVEN does not account for my feelings, orientatory inclinations, or manners of relational world-making. I do not necessarily believe that I was born asexual but rather that I have asexual tendencies, that I came into asexuality in the way I came into queerness: because it provided me with meaningful self-narratives and held open theoretical, activist, and erotic possibilities. Asexual, as much as queer, can gesture toward "the open mesh of possibilities, gaps, overlaps, dissonances and resonances," drawing on Eve Kosofsky Sedgwick's memorable words, that challenge sexual categorization.[6] In this sense, *Asexual Erotics* is written from a place that is invested in asexual visibility and yet leaves me sometimes fraught at writing a book that is less about an identity and more about critiquing sexually overdetermined modes of relating.

In what follows of the introduction, I provide a frame for thinking about asexuality and erotics. First, I provide a brief introduction to interdisciplinary work on asexuality by highlighting how asexual activism, asexuality in the health sciences, and feminist and queer approaches to asexuality approach definitions of asexuality. Next, I explore "erotics," drawing on Audre Lorde's reimagining of this Platonian and Freudian concept, to deepen our understanding of intimacy and relating and offer a meaningful language for thinking about the coordinates of asexuality.[7] In the final portion of the introduction, I unpack the chapters in the book, discussing them as a series of "intimate readings," a series of asexually driven analyses of feminist, queer, and lesbian cultures, that foster an expansive approach to both asexuality and erotics.

## THINKING ASEXUALITY (IN AT LEAST THREE VOICES): ACTIVISMS, SCIENCES, AND QUEER FEMINISMS

### *Defining Asexuality, Redefining Sexuality: Asexual Activisms and Countercultures*

The sexual identity and orientation of asexuality has a rich cultural, historical, and political life, even as it continues to be overlooked and neglected in LGBTQ2+ (lesbian, gay, bisexual, transgender, queer, two-spirit, plus) spaces and narratives. While asexuality is commonly understood as not being sexually attracted to others, the very modes of defining it are nuanced and contested. Online asexual communities include the online platform AVEN, as well as blogs and social networking sites such as Reddit and Tumblr. Offline, asexual organizing happens locally and internationally, including through meet-ups, conferences, pride parades, zine publications, and an annual "Asexual Awareness Week" (held in the last week of October).[8] AVEN, in particular, is an online community and education space of deep value and meaning. Launched by asexual activist David Jay in 2001, it now includes over 250,000 members (as of January 1, 2017) and provides a space for asexually identified people (also known as "aces") to meet outside of mainstream sexual society as well as to address the invisibility of and discrimination against asexual people through education and awareness.[9] AVEN's creation marks a landmark moment for asexuality because it provides the language for thinking of asexuality as a sexual orientation and identity, drawing on the vocabulary of sexual orientation models. By using the language of "sexual attraction," asexuality is granted visibility alongside other sexual orientations that likewise pivot the criterion of "sexual attraction."[10] In this sense, by articulating an absence of a desire for sex and an absence of sexual attraction, asexual voices demonstrate that asexuality is thinkable within the modern regime of sexuality. This articulation of asexuality along lines of sexual attraction is an important political move in terms of visibility and education, as it allows for asexuality to be mapped onto already existing understandings of how sexual identities and orientations operate within common understandings of sexuality.

Yet even prior to AVEN, asexuality as a nameable sexual orientation was articulated and formulated, including on the internet. Jay, AVEN's founder, indicates that through comments on boards unrelated to asexuality, early message boards, and Zoe O'Reilly's blog post "My Life as an Amoeba" (1997), early "proto-identity" took form, leading to Jay's launch of AVEN.[11] Reilly (1997), for instance, called for "the world to know that we are out there," stimulating responses from many other asexual people and the creation of the Yahoo! Group "The Haven for the Human Amoeba" (2000).[12]

While asexual activist definitions often draw on the concept of "sexual attraction," they also trouble it. Definitions of asexuality springing from the asexual, or ace, community suggest that sexual attraction is not an innate aspect of intimate or interpersonal life, thus challenging compulsory sexuality or the belief that sex and sexuality are core components of being human. Challenging the idea that everyone is sexual, ace online and offline communities also generate other vocabularies and understandings of thinking about attraction and sexuality. Importantly, romantic and aromantic are vital qualifiers within ace communities, contributing another axis to how we imagine attraction between individuals. Aromantic individuals are colloquially known as "aros" and aromanticism indicates a low interest in romantic contact as well as a prioritizing of friendship, or of being "friend-focused."[13] Aromantic identity troubles "amatonormativity," or the organization of life and love according to a hierarchy that prioritizes sexual and romantic couples.[14] Romantic asexuality includes an interest in building romantic, if not sex-based, relationships with others, which may include kissing, touching, and cuddling. Other attractional modes that are explored by asexual communities on- and offline include *aesthetic* attraction ("attraction to someone's appearance") and *sensual* attraction ("desire to have physical non-sexual contact with someone else, like affectionate touching").[15]

*Romantic* and *aromantic* are also relevant descriptors for people who are not asexual, as they help to grasp an aspect of the manner in which people are attracted to each other, rather than assuming that attraction relies only upon the desire to have sex. These conceptual contributions by asexual communities build on decades of queer work toward understanding how what are commonly called "sexual identities" as well as "orientations" hold entire worlds of possibilities within them even as they reduce these possibilities to one-word labels such as "lesbian," "gay," "bisexual," "pansexual," and "asexual." Sedgwick, in particular, questioned what gets condensed into sexual identities, providing a dynamic list ranging from one's own gender identity, the gender of the recipient of one's attraction, sexual acts, fantasies, emotional bonds, power, and community.[16] Thus, sexual identities are formulaic labels that exist within the modern regime of sexuality and glaze over most aspects of relating, including the many possible manners of attraction and the practices they generate. Yet, because of the central role that sex has played within determining sexual identity, sexual identity has been understood as based on *sexual* attraction—or the idea that it is the desire to have sex with someone that is the key deciding factor of which sexual identity one classifies as, rendering other forms of attraction "nondiactrical differences," in Sedgwick's words.[17] As attraction has been reduced to sexual attraction, so sexual identities and orientations have been understood as resting on both the gender of who we are purportedly drawn to and the desire to be sexual.[18] Asexual elaborations of other forms of attraction implicitly question the basis of grounding identities and orientations in sexual desire, thereby also questioning, more broadly, modern systems of sexuality that have been taking shape since the late seventeenth century in Western settler contexts.[19] Importantly, systems of sexuality that have been developed to categorize people into sexual personas have historically functioned as systems of colonial imposition underwritten by desires to keep heterosexuality tethered to whiteness, normality, and ability.[20] Asexual communities' careful explorations of what constitutes attraction in the first place point to the importance of seeing sex and sexuality as bound yet separate concepts: bound because sexual desire underwrites the system of sexuality and separate because asexuality, even as it signifies an absence or low level of sexual attraction, can nonetheless be formulated within the parameters of what we know of as "sexuality." In turn, asexuality, as much as all sexual inclinations and practices, is both bolstered by sexuality, as we know it, and hampered by it—leading to the emergence of a sexual identity that until very recently was thought impossible even as it is evidently present throughout the history of modern sexuality.

Asexual organizing also presents opportunities for spectrum- and umbrella-based approaches to asexual identification that draw on Kinseyian ideas of orientation as based on degrees rather than fixed points. Alfred Kinsey outlined a model for thinking sexual orientation based on the degree to which one was attracted to one gender or another (with gender understood on a binary model), demonstrating the extent to which most people fall within the bisexual range.[21] Asexual communities draw on this spectrum concept to put forward additional forms of spectrum-based identification, including a romantic-aromantic axis as well as a sexual-asexual axis. "Gray asexuality," or "gray-A," thus refers to people who fall on the asexual end of the sexual-asexual axis, including those who are asexually identified yet who sometimes experience sexual attraction to others. "Demi-sexual," in turn, refers to people who experience sexual attraction to those they are intimately bonded with first. Figure 0.1b, from the widely circulated zine by Maisha, *Taking the Cake: An Illustrated Primer on Asexuality* (for the cover, see figure 0.1a), expertly portrays the many possible jars of ingredients that go into making asexual identity labels. As Maisha outlines, these include aromantic, ace, demisexual, heteroromantic (being romantically attracted to the opposite gender), homoromantic (being romantically attracted to the same gender), grey asexuality (or gray asexuality), repulsed (as in repulsed by sex), indifferent (as in indifferent to sex), panromantic (being romantically attracted to all genders), and biromantic (being romantically attracted to two genders). These "flavors" challenge the idea that there is only one way to be asexual and that a single definition of asexuality can function to explain people's unique engagements with asexuality across social contexts.[22] Further, spectrum labels such as "gray-A" present opportunities for troubling a stark division between people who are "sexual" and "asexual" because they challenge the sexual presumption, or the idea that being sexual is the default and neutral mode of being. As asexual writer Julie Sondra Decker indicates, another term that challenges the

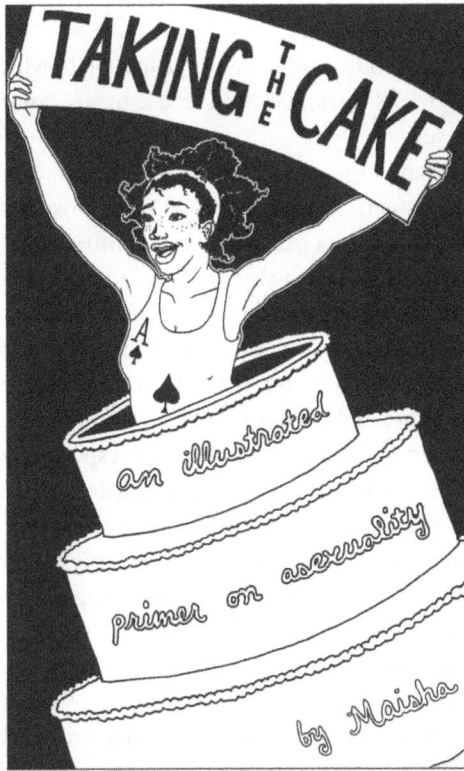

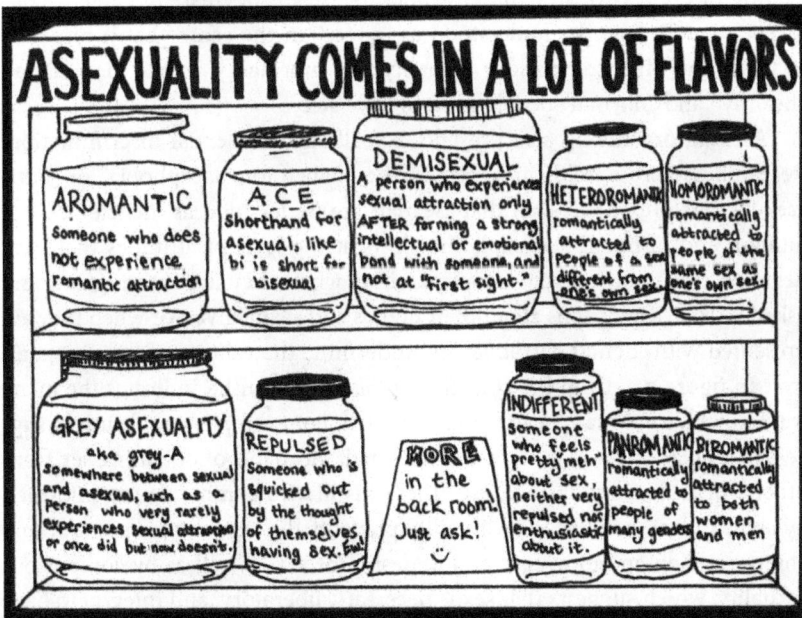

**FIGURE 0.1A AND 0.1B.** From the zine *Taking the Cake: An Illustrated Primer on Asexuality* by Maisha, 2012. The zine is available online at https://acezinearchive.wordpress.com/ace-zine-list/101-informational-zines/taking-the-cake-an-illustrated-primer-on-asexuality/.[23]

assumed neutrality around being sexual is "allosexual," which, derived from "alloerotic" in Sedgwick's work, has been in use by ace communities to refer to people who are sexual.[24]

Ace community and organizing also stresses the importance of envisioning asexual identity as part of queer and LGBTQ2+ organizing. Asexuality is an orientation that cuts across other sexual identities, such that in addition to identifying as asexual, aces will also identify as bisexual, lesbian, gay, pansexual, and straight, as well as monogamous and polyamorous and romantic and aromantic. Many asexually identified individuals fall under the transgender umbrella and are transmasculine, transfeminine, trans men, trans women, genderqueer, nonbinary, and agender. According to the 2014 Asexual Community Census, only 75 percent of the 10,880 ace respondents who completed the survey identified categorically as "woman/female" or "man/male."[25] These numbers have also been triangulated by academic research. For example, one study found that of sixty-six asexual participants eighteen chose identities that were nonbinary, including gender-neutral, androgynous, or genderqueer.[26] This overlap between queer, trans, and asexual is important to remember since many asexual people report feeling excluded from queer and LGBTQ2+ spaces.[27] Further, if we think of queerness as not only a matter of gender of object choice but also one of non-normative intimacies and the political challenging of oppressive straight, cisgender, racist, misogynist, and ableist contexts, asexuality can be understood as "queer" in the sense that it responds to ideas that bind compulsory sexuality with normality, or the idea that all "healthy" and "normal" people need to have sex.

Asexual organizing also presents a challenge to asexual discrimination. Researchers across fields have provided evidence for "asexphobia" or "anti-asexual bias/prejudice" such that asexuals are understood as "deficient," "less human, and disliked."[28] Asexphobia exists at the level of attitudes that have negative effects on asexual people such as when they are interrogated and asked intrusive questions about their bodies and sexual lives, or when they are presented with "denial narratives" to undermine the validity of their asexuality.[29] In figure 0.2, from the zine *Taking the Cake*, Maisha indicates the many ways in which asexuality can be undermined. For example, people might suggest that an ace person is repressed, closeted, incapable of obtaining sex from others, or in an immature phase. These dismissive comments are informed by ableist ideas, such as that disability prevents the capacity for sex and that ability rests on an enjoyment of and desire for sex as well as by compulsory sexuality, which suggests that sex is necessary, liberatory, and integral to happiness and well-being. Discrimination can also take on the form of social and sexual exclusion, including in queer contexts: through "conversion" practices

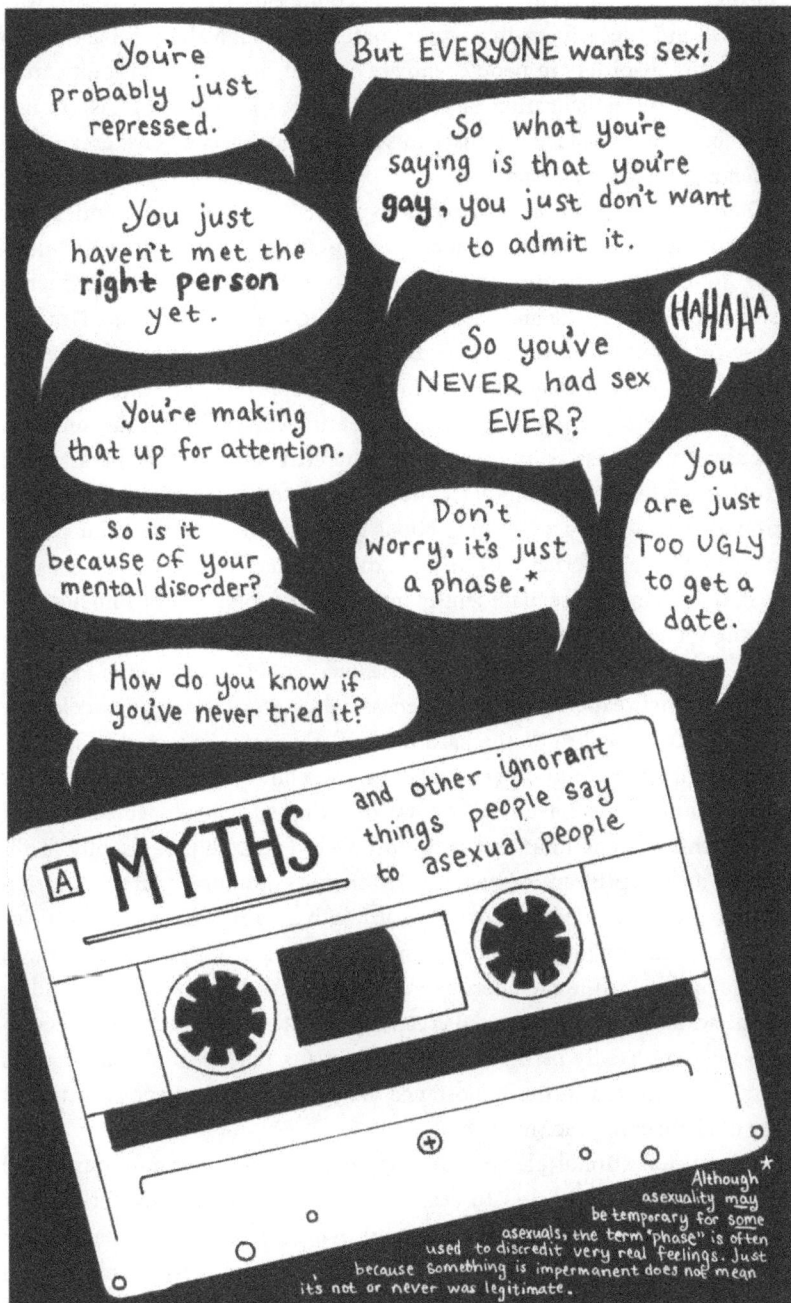

**FIGURE 0.2.** A selection of "denial narratives." From *Taking the Cake: An Illustrated Primer on Asexuality* zine by Maisha, 2012.[30]

in medical and clinical environments to encourage asexuals to have sex, with unwanted and coerced sex in partner contexts, through the misdiagnosis of sexual desire disorders in people who are asexual, and with invisibility, toxic attention, or the fetishization of asexual identity.[31] Recognizing discrimination is important because it refuses to see individual acts against asexuals as incidental, providing a systemic view on patterns of "dislike" against asexuals.

Yet even as asexuals experience "asexphobia," asexual communities tend to be white-dominated spaces that are not immune to racism. As contributors of the *Brown and Gray* zine point out, aces of color often feel isolated when raising questions of race and asexuality in white-dominated spaces. Drawing on one contributor to the zine, asexuality is often imagined as a "white orientation—an identity that belong[s] to white people only" in ways that make asexuality difficult for people of color to identify with and that draw on racist ideas about whiteness as inherently sexually reticent against the backdrop of "sexualized others."[32] As another contributor to the zine writes, "When I'm surrounded by white aces, talking about race is hard."[33] Ace of color people also speak to the experience of being sexualized in a way that white aces are not, so that claiming asexual identity for people of color can be difficult, and they might be met with additional undermining comments such as that they do not "look asexual." Further, white asexual people are not often expected to speak to their experiences of whiteness, while asexual people of color are routinely called upon to do the hard work of "race talk" in regard to asexuality. To address these and other effects of racism and foster antiracism, many asexual communities have moved toward having spaces for people of color only, yet this is sometimes met with pushback. For example, recently facilitating a workshop in an asexual and aromantic community on white privilege, our group decided to move forward with creating an ace/aro of color meet-up. While the majority of the community was in support of this move, a couple of vocal white members expressed strong feelings of being excluded, and one white member suggested creating a "white-only" meet-up as recompense for purportedly being excluded, suggesting that asexual communities are unevenly alerted to the importance of struggles around social justice in terms of challenging racism.

A final definitional element arising from asexual communities is the idea of different approaches to sex and sexuality. Sociologist Mark Carrigan observed that there are three general dynamics among asexual people: sex positivity, sex neutrality, and sex repulsion.[34] In this sense, some asexual people experience repulsion to sex, while others "love that you love sex"—as David Jay shouted to onlookers at a San Francisco pride parade featured in the documentary *(A)sexual* (2011).[35] In figure 0.1b, by Maisha, both repulsed and indifferent are illustrated as flavors that constitute asexual identity, suggesting the importance of recognizing divergent approaches to sex within asexual communities. Further, some asexual people engage in sex and BDSM, suggesting that sexual behavior and sexual identity are not always linked in obvious or absolute ways.[36] It is significant to understand all these positionalities as valid and as part of the spectrum of approaches to asexuality and sexuality more broadly. Because of the many aspects and types of asexual identification and experiences, as listed above, it is useful to think of asexuality in the plural as "asexualities"—an intricate identity that is not possible to contain within one definition.[37]

## From Pathology to Allyhood: Science and Asexuality

In distinction to asexual communities, scientific researchers of the past and present tend to take on different approaches to measuring and defining asexualities. Sometimes functioning as asexual allies and other times pathologizing asexuality, health and medical scientific researchers strive to use the measures, tools, languages, and methods of science to demonstrate how sexual orientations, including asexuality, operate in the body and mind, as well as to quantify the occurrence of asexuality among the general population.

Historically, there has been a host of diagnoses that pathologized low levels of sexual desire. Low sexual desire has, since the nineteenth century, been captured with such terms as "sexual anesthesia," "sexual coldness," frigidity, and "inhibited sexual desire," and more recently as "hypoactive sexual desire disorder" and within the *Diagnostic and Statistical Manual of Mental Disorders, 5th Edition (DSM-V)* as "female sexual interest/arousal disorder" and "male hypoactive sexual desire disorder."[38] These labels have functioned mostly to problematize women's (and primarily white women's) low levels of sexual desire disproportionately. It has been argued that with the turn of the twentieth century, discourses of white women's "passionlessness" or their presumed innate low sexual desire began to shift to ideas that women were meant to be—within the proper heterosexual and marital context—sexual and sexually desiring.[39] Further, this increase in the preferred level of white women's sexual desire in the early twentieth century is tied also to a fear that whiteness was under threat due to a lower birth rate, motivating a new intoxication with marriage as a site of sexual satisfaction for white women and a move away from their previously purported "asexual" nature.[40]

Alfred Kinsey's development of the seven-point scale of sexual orientation in the 1940s and 1950s provided an early example of scientific conceptualizations of asexuality. While it is well known that Kinsey stipulated a spectrum-based model of hetero-homo attraction, what is less known is that he also put forward a category known as group "X," which he understood as including those with "no socio-sexual contacts or reactions," and who "do not respond erotically to either heterosexual or homosexual stimuli, and do not have overt physical contacts with individuals of either sex in which there is evidence of any response."[41] Further, Kinsey identified 2 percent of men over twenty-five and "a goodly number of females" as belonging to this group.[42] It is interesting to note that asexuality, in Kinsey's model, occupied a space outside of the hetero-homo spectrum, placing asexuals as outliers on the map of sexual orientation.

Michael Storms's work from the late 1970s and early 1980s provided the next major engagement with asexuality through a reconceptualization of Kinsey's scale in the form of a four-quadrant grid that includes not only heterosexuality and homosexuality but also bisexuality and asexuality, each with a quarter of the grid space.[43] Notably, Storms, along with similar work by Paula Nurius, provided a first articulation of asexuality by seeing asexuality as a sexual orientation.[44] Further, William Masters, Virginia Johnson, and Robert Kolodny provided some recognition of asexuality in their "typology of homosexuals," discussing "asexual homosexuals" as "low in sexual interest and activity and . . . not 'coupled.'"[45] They identified 16 percent of gay men and 11 percent of lesbians as asexual. Unfortunately, in the process of identifying gay asexuality, they also pathologized asexuals by rendering them "more secretive," "dysfunctional," "worse off psychologically" than other homosexuals, and "generally loners."[46]

A groundbreaking piece of scientific scholarship on asexuality came in 2004 when Anthony Bogaert published an analysis of the preexisting UK National Survey of Sexual Attitudes and Lifestyles (1994), which happened to have as one of its answer choices "I have never felt sexually attracted to anyone at all."[47] Bogaert's seminal piece, invested in deducing whether or not asexuality was "real," brought scientific and popular attention to asexuality in an unprecedented way. After its publication, many mainstream popular news sources and talk shows, including Fox News, The View, Montel Williams, ABC's 20/20, and CNN, did specials on asexuality, inviting AVEN's David Jay, other asexually identified individuals, "(s)experts" such as sex counselors and scientific sex researchers, and Bogaert himself to speak on behalf of the legitimacy of asexuality. While lending visibility to asexuality, much of this popular attention functioned to spectacularize and fetishize asexuals while also representing those who are mostly white and able-bodied, and over-representing cisgender male asexuals as exemplars of asexuality.[48]

Bogaert's operationalization of asexuality in both his 2004 piece as well as in his other work, such as his book, tends to provide a limiting definition of asexuality that treats asexuals as objects of research to be studied.[49] Yet a major benefit of Bogaert's study was that it presented a quantitative indication of what percentage of the population might be asexual that has since been used to add legitimacy and credibility to asexuality both in research and the media. Bogaert's 2004 study presents us with a 1.05 percent of the population as asexual, while other studies have ranged from 0.4 to 5.5 percent.[50] It is important to note the Western focus of these studies as well as that they tend to draw on preexisting data.[51]

Contemporary scientific research on asexuality focuses on exploring subjective versus physiological arousal, while for the most part arguing against understandings of asexuality as a pathology. Most prominently, Lori Brotto and colleagues at the UBC Sexual Health Lab have undertaken studies to ascertain that asexuality is a sexual orientation (as opposed to a paraphilia or a sexual dysfunction) and to establish how it is possible for physiological/genital arousal to be present even as subjective attraction is not.[52] Brotto and colleagues have also developed an "Asexuality Identification Scale," which consists of twelve questions that measure whether someone is asexual through asking whether the person has experienced sexual attraction, whether an ideal relationship for them would involve sexual activity, and whether they avoid situations that might include sex.[53]

Brotto, alongside asexual activists such as David Jay and Andrew Hinderliter, played a key role in removing asexuality as a sexual disorder from the *Diagnostic and Statistical Manual,* such that the *DSM-V* now has exceptions for asexuality under low sexual desire diagnoses. Further, whereas the *DSM-IV* articulated so-called interpersonal distress as a proper cause for diagnosing hypoactive sexual desire disorder (HSDD), the *DSM-V* does not allow interpersonal distress to be an indicator of female sexual interest/arousal disorder (FSIAD) or male hypoactive sexual desire disorder (MHSDD), protecting asexual people from being pathologized due to distress that may result from partners having asymmetrical desires and expectations around sex.[54] Notably, there is a politics and money-generating factor at work in these diagnoses, especially with the US Food and Drug Administration (FDA) approval of the drug Flibanserin/Addyi for the treatment of HSDD/FSIAD in 2015, which despite unimpressive clinical trials can now be prescribed to cisgender women as a Viagra equivalent for stimulating sexual desire.

Health scientific and medical scientific research on asexuality has a checkered relationship with asexuality, much as with other sexual orientations. With the "truth-based" quality often granted to scientific and medical knowledge, it often tends to function as the final word on asexuality and its definitions. While there are possibilities and examples of allyship and of adding legitimacy to asexuality, scientific research can also easily pathologize asexuality because of its commitment to the wedding of "health" and "normality" with sexual desire and attraction through an investment in compulsory sexuality. More broadly, because scientific approaches to studying sexual identities are deeply invested in sexuality as an organizing set of discourses for how the self is understood, these approaches often play a central role in entrenching sex, even if they create exceptions for asexuality.

### Resonances and Intersectionality: Queer and Feminist Approaches to Defining Asexuality

Throughout this book, I hone a queer and feminist approach to asexuality that challenges the pathologization and invisibilization of asexuality. In doing so, I draw on the energies of what has emerged as a feminist and queer approach to asexuality and the inventive and collaborative work of gender and sexuality studies scholars who have been thinking about asexuality for nearing on the last decade. Queer and feminist approaches to asexuality bring with them a unique set of contributions to both asexuality and to gender and sexuality studies, challenging, as I explore below, both compulsory sexuality and essentialist approaches to asexuality.

First, queer and feminist approaches to asexuality tend to both broaden and pluralize what can "count" as asexuality and how asexuality is defined. KJ Cerankowski and M. Milks have written that by calling attention to the plural embodiments and expressions of asexuality as asexualities in the plural, we can more fully account for the spectrum of asexual experiences.[55] With Danielle Cooper, I build on this analysis by calling for a broadening of definitions of asexuality.[56] Instead of accepting the definitions of asexuality put forward by the "truth archive" of science, we invite an understanding of "asexual resonances" that challenges the assumption that queerness must be sexual in nature, asserting that "where there is queerness there is also asexuality."[57] Broadening and pluralizing asexual definitions is important because it is both a more inclusive approach to asexuality and also one that acknowledges sexual fluidity—or that a/sexuality changes over the course of a lifespan. This presents a direct challenge to some of the more limiting understandings of asexuality, such as psychologist Anthony Bogaert's assertion that asexuality, in order to count as an orientation, must be lifelong, or the *DSM-V*'s commentary that for women to not be diagnosed with female sexual interest/arousal disorder, they must have never experienced sexual attraction.[58] In this sense, feminist and queer approaches to asexuality push back against a medical model that tends to pathologize low sexual desire.

Second, feminist and queer broadenings of definitions around asexuality also constitute an expansion of the asexual archive, challenging what has tended to be a cisgender, male, and white canon of asexuality. Canonized examples of asexuality include characters and representations such as Todd  Chavez on *BoJack Horseman,* Jughead Jones in the comic series *Archie, Doctor Who,* Sheldon Cooper on *The Big Bang Theory,* Sherlock Holmes, and the first asexual character featured on mainstream TV, Gerald Tippett, on the New Zealand soap opera *Shortland Street.* Broadening the archive around asexuality involves thinking about asexuality intersectionally, questioning why asexuality can only "count" if it is a born-this-way type of sexual orientation, allowing for (a)sexual fluidity over the lifespan, and focusing on queer and feminist representations of asexuality in particular.[59] For example, Eunjung Kim compellingly expands the asexual archive by focusing on asexuality and disability in Donna Williams's memoirs about her experiences with autism and asexuality and in the film *Snow Cake* (2006), which also features an autistic and asexual character.[60] Through doing this, she challenges the able-bodied canon of asexuality that is invested in proving that asexuals are "normal" and not "disabled." In a different way, with Cooper, I situate the artist Agnes Martin and writer Valerie Solanas as "asexual" in a broad sense of the term, suggesting that an asexual art practice and political asexuality, respectively, can be other modes through which to understand asexuality in conversation with asexual orientation and in contexts of compulsory sexuality.[61]

Third, queer and feminist approaches to asexuality also place asexuality in direct dialogue with larger power structures and patterns of injustice. The concept of compulsory sexuality, in particular, has been a central contribution of growing asexuality studies research. As a term, it draws on Adrienne Rich's "compulsory *heterosexuality*" to index the ways in which sexuality, like heterosexuality, is assumed to be original, primary, prevalent, preferred, and superior, and thus socially rewarded and bolstered, to the detriment of other sexualities.[62] Developing the term "compulsory sexuality" by drawing on the work of legal scholar Elizabeth Emens, Kristina Gupta elaborates on the ways in which compulsory sexuality is a system that encourages some people to have sex, even while banning marginalized groups from sexual expression through the process of "desexualization."[63] Desexualization, as Kim's work explores, functions to render marginalized groups such as people with disabilities, lesbians and transgender people, children and older adults, people of size, and some racialized people as "asexual" by default—misusing the term "asexuality" in the process.[64] Desexualization ranges from discourses around people with disabilities not being capable of sex or not being desirable to eugenics-based initiatives for managing a population through controlling reproduction by methods of coerced sterilization.

Desexualization and compulsory sexuality are also linked to hypersexualization, or the branding of some groups—most especially gay men and racialized groups—as excessively sexual and lascivious and thus in need of "population management." Treatment of people with AIDS in the 1980s, for example, and the pivoting of the "AIDS epidemic" as "God's punishment for being gay" demonstrates how the deployment of hypersexualization, in combination with homophobia, can have lethal effects on marginalized communities.[65] Lauren Berlant and Lee Edelman wrote that "heteronormativity attempts to snuff out libidinal unruliness by projecting evidence of it onto . . . other populations deemed excessively appetitive," demonstrating how queer people can easily become hypersexualized in aggressive and life-threatening ways.[66] Ianna Hawkins Owen discusses how compulsory sexuality has uneven racial histories, such that whiteness has tended to emulate an "asexuality-as-ideal" as demonstrative of a form of innocence, moral control, and restraint, while black people have often been positioned as hypersexual so as to justify enslavement, lynching, and other instruments of racism.[67] Hypersexualization and desexualization have thus been used historically and are in the present used as forms of social control and oppression, and toward the maintenance of a white, able-bodied, heteropatriarchal nation-state. So while it is fair to argue that sex, under the modern regime of sexuality, is encouraged, compulsory sexuality also rests on the white, ableist, and heteronormative hope and expectation that some people will *not* have sex, with the implementation of tactics for curtailing sex for those deemed dangerous to a nation-state: gay people, queer people, people of color, disabled people. This uneven application of compulsory sexuality takes shape differently across social groups such that histories of desexualization and hypersexualization are highly specific and varied. What is important is that the terminology around compulsory sexuality reminds us that "appropriate" and "normal" levels of desire are always caught up in discourses around gender, race, ability, and sexual orientation. Feminist and queer research on asexuality thus invites examinations of the intersectional histories and present-day realities of compulsory sexuality.

Fourth, feminist and queer researchers have also situated asexuality as a possible mode of resistance against oppressive social structures. Asexuality, in this sense, is explored less as a sexual orientation than as a political strategy. Breanne Fahs explored asexuality as a "radical refusal" in use by women's liberation feminists such as Cell 16, Dana Densmore and Roxanne Dunbar-Ortiz (members of Cell 16), and Valerie Solanas.[68] In various ways, these feminists articulated a refusal of sex, and particularly heterosexual sex, as a means of getting things done in the women's revolution, creating world systems apart from cisgender men, and exploring various forms of erotics between women. Asexuality was likewise articulated as both an antisexist and antiracist strategy by figures such as writer Toni Cade Bambara and the Puerto Rican group the National Young Lords Party (YLP), as I will explore in the first chapter. Bambara articulates sex as a colonial form of control against black women, while the women of the YLP staged a sex strike in 1970 as a way to demand that changes be made within the party, such as elevating women to positions of power, eradicating machismo, and educating the group on feminist concerns.[69] Through situating political asexuality as a form of sex rebellion, these and other feminists provided an oppositional platform to racism, sexism, and patriarchy, as well as to ideas of compulsory sexuality or "sexusociety"—a society organized around sex.[70]

To best illustrate some of the key contributions of a queer and feminist approach to asexuality studies, I want to briefly demonstrate how these perspectives lend themselves to unpacking representations of asexuality in mainstream media.[71] In a portrayal of asexuality on an episode of Fox network's medical drama *House,* which originally aired on January 23, 2012 ("Better Half"), a white, young, attractive, presumably able-bodied, heterosexual, married, and asexual couple enters the doctor's office (see figures 0.3a and b). Getting caught in the orbit of Dr. Greg House (played by Hugh Laurie) and his team of doctors due to a simple bladder infection, the couple become promptly suspect in their asexuality and subject to a series of medical tests. As the episode unfolds, and Dr. House persists in his disbelief of asexuality, asexuality continues to be undermined, erased, and misrepresented on two fronts. While the husband is found to have a tumor on his pituitary gland that caused his asexuality, his partner is found to be lying about her asexuality so as to make her husband happy. Though the couple has been together and asexual for ten years, *House* teaches its audience that their asexuality is impossible. In the words of Dr. House, we learn only that sex is "the fundamental drive of our species, sex is healthy" and that "the only people who don't want it are either sick, dead, or lying."[72]

Mobilizing feminist and queer approaches to asexuality provides the possibility for recognizing the harmful and undermining aspects of this representation, while also assessing how it reproduces asexuality on terms tied to whiteness, normativity, heterosexuality, and able-bodiedness. First, drawing on queer and feminist affirmations of asexuality, it is possible to question why asexuality is rendered impossible in this scenario—that is because compulsory sexuality renders sexual behavior necessary for all subjects deemed "capable" of it. Asexuality is represented as impossible, as a fabrication, and as a problem to be resolved. *House*'s pernicious portrayal of asexuality effectively renders the social expectation that sex is a universal norm and obligation that

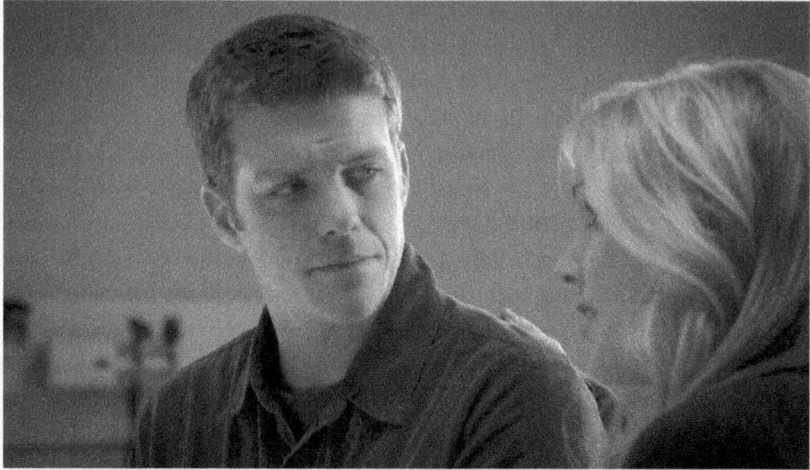

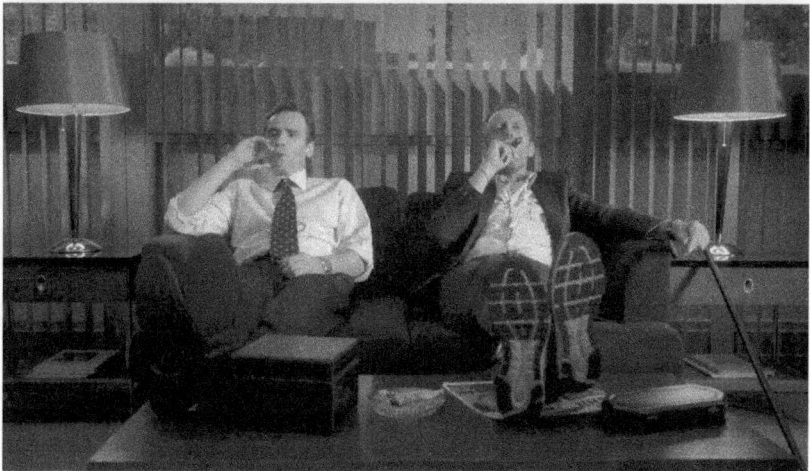

**FIGURES 0.3A AND 0.3B.** Asexuality on Fox Network's *House*; the episode "Better Half" originally aired on January 23, 2012. The first image is of the couple learning that a brain tumor has led to asexuality in the man and that the woman is lying about asexuality. The second image is of the doctors reclining and sharing a cigar after their findings.

is entangled with whiteness, youth, normativity, able-bodiedness, coupling, and heterosexuality. It suggests that physiologically rooted asexuality is itself invalid as a sexual identity. Low levels of sexual desire are problematized by *House* as impossible and unfathomable without a medial cause, which, once found, opens the door to the practice of healthful coupled sex. *House* implies that it is indeed certain types of bodies that are encouraged to be sexual and desire sex and that to not be sexual or desire sex is inherently wrong and in need of fixing.

Drawing on intersectional approaches to asexuality, it is possible to observe the degree to which whiteness is implicated here along with compulsory sexuality, heterosexuality, and ability. As with the whiteness of the couple, the space of medical science in this representation is likewise primarily white as well as mostly male and cisgender. White male doctors are shown as scientific researchers who move across spaces of privilege with ease and in suits, digging deep into a person's body through the use of a laboratory and its feminized lab assistants. Indeed, sex surfaces here as an obligation for hetero-coupled subjects under projects of white supremacist race preservation, monitored and encouraged at the hands of white doctors.[73] *House* suggests that even as asexuality is unimaginable, it still is most easily framed through whiteness as whiteness gone awry. While sexual reticence has been discursively viewed as an achievement of whiteness, as Hawkins Owen and Julian Carter both discuss, white asexuality is nonetheless framed as a wasted whiteness. In ways parallel to the mourning of white, attractive, able-bodied gay men and women by heterosexuality, the white asexual individual is mourned as a wasted and wasteful whiteness because of its oblique relationship to heterosexual compulsory sexuality. Drawing on the words of Julian Carter, the white asexual couple is seen as "wast[ing] the productive potential of [their] bod[ies] as a vector for the transmission of whiteness to the next generation" by not engaging in sex, sexual reproduction, and sexual desire.[74] Queer and feminist approaches to this representation thus demand an intersectionally grounded suspicion in how asexuality is rendered impossible. Further, a credulous approach to writing off asexuality because it is the result of pathology, as Dr. House deduces, challenges medical science as the final authority on how people can make meanings of their sexual identities and relational lives.

Asexuality, like any other sexual orientation, is widely varied in terms of experiences, intersecting identities, and expressions. Health and medical scientific research has seesawed between pathologizing asexuality and legitimating it as a sexual orientation, whereas feminist and queer researchers have explored the political, intersectional, and resistance-based possibilities of asexuality, questioning limiting definitions of asexuality and asking that asexuality be thought alongside desexualization. Asexual activists and community members, as history makers of the asexuality movement, have provided online and offline languages, vocabularies, and symbologies around asexuality, arguing for its inclusion in LGBTQ2+ spaces, bringing asexuality into visibility in unprecedented ways. Together, the overlapping spaces of research and activism question asexual omissions in queer spaces and stories and compel us to think about sexual orientation and identity beyond sexual attraction.

## AN EROTIC FRAMEWORK

Drawing on the interdisciplinary work outlined above, this book argues that asexuality is an unmined provocation of erotic possibilities, a theoretical, affective, and relational challenge to imagining what can be. Susie Scott and Matt Dawson offer the observation that research on asexuality has tended to prioritize asexual people as atomistic units instead of thinking about them in contexts of relating.[75] Parallel to this analysis, according to Staci Newmahr, insufficient research has explored "eroticism in its own right, distinct from sexual behaviors and identities."[76] *Erotics* thus provide a promising language for discussing forms of intimacy that are simply not reducible to sex and sexuality and that, further, challenge the Freudian doxa that the sexual is at the base of all things.

Erotics derive from the Ancient Greek *eros*, which was understood by Plato to be one form of love among many, including friendship love and familial love, but which was arguably not bound to sexual passion.[77] In *Symposium*, eros surfaces as a love for the good, a desire for immortality—a mytho-spiritual plane touching with but not bound to sexuality.[78] But then in Sigmund Freud's work, eros became bound strongly to sexual passion through the assertion that the sexual drive and libido are at the base of all human action and relationships—at the base of all erotics.[79] Yet even Freud himself admitted that "it is not easy to decide what is covered by the concept 'sexual.'"[80] Arguing against the restriction of sexuality to sex itself, Freud expanded the horizon of "sexuality" or "the sexual" beyond adult heterosexuality. By provocatively muddying up the separation between sexual love and "nonsexual" love, Freud's lifetime of work argued that sexuality is, essentially, at the base of much love and action—starting with child-parent relations, including samesex attraction, and through to the "sublimation" of the sexual instinct into creative action in the world. Further, even nonsexual action becomes "sexual" such that an absence of a sex drive (or asexuality) is understood as "repression" of one's sexual instincts.[81] The absence and excess of a sexual desire in women through frigidity, hysteria, and neuroses—which we could loosely term as historical resonances of asexuality—are foundational moments for psychoanalysis. Asexuality, the lack of sexual drive or desire, as well as hypersexuality, a deemed excessiveness of sexual desire, especially when found in women, became key informants within the formation of Freudian psychoanalysis. Importantly, through the Freudian tradition, *eros* came to be understood as rooted in "the sexual" and framed as a sexual life force and libidinal energy behind all human progress, action, and "civilization" itself.[82] Following on Freud, erotics have become popularly conflated with the sex drive, with sexual desire, and more broadly with muddy understandings of sexuality in general.[83]

Yet erotics for feminists, and for my own work in particular, are about challenging the conflation of sexual desire with the erotic and thus opening up different paradigms for thinking about relating. Writing on Plato and Freud, Stella Sandford argues that "eros, in all its manifestations, is neither somatic nor psychical, neither 'sexual' nor 'non-sexual,' but both," providing an avenue into understanding how erotics is not only an appropriate but an ideal term for conceptualizing asexuality.[84] Queer feminist Lynne Huffer explores how the language of erotics and eros seems to make possible a different analysis than a focus on "sexuality" permits, suggesting a break from a biopolitical sexuality and an attempt to think intimacy in a way that is not affixed to neoliberal modes of relating.[85] She writes that "eros is the name we can give to a mode of living . . . [that is] an uncertain, embodied, disruptive encounter of subjects with others," productively centering eros and erotic engagement over sexuality.[86] Drawing on Huffer and on a Foucauldian tradition, I understand sexuality as a system for categorizing desire that arose as part and parcel of capitalism, modernity, and colonialism. As such, sexuality is a technique of biopower that invents normalcy and deviancy toward forwarding the interests of colonialism, whiteness, wealth, ability, and normality, at the expense of sexuality's "others" including its colonized subjects, people of color, poor people, disabled people, and those understood as sexually "deviant." Grounded in Darwinian evolutionary theories, the development of sexuality as a series of theories of the body is at its heart about reproducing the "fit" and preventing the "unfit" from reproducing, and through this managing the population.[87] As such, the invention of elaborate techniques and forms of knowledge have encouraged health and sex among some while discouraging, including through desexualization and hypersexualization, health and sex among others. Sex has thus been encouraged within sexuality as compulsory with the implicit understanding that some people's desires for sex must be kept in check, must be studied, ordered, exploited, and categorized to preserve common interests of whiteness and morality. If sexuality is harnessed in this way by biopolitics toward the regimentation and disciplining of bodies, the reproduction of the health of the population, rendering sex compulsory for some (through compulsory sexuality) and banning it for others (through desexualization), then eros and the erotic can be seen as hoping for another tradition of thinking desire.[88]

In using the language of "erotics," I draw on a feminist, lesbian, and antiracist lineage. Most notably, in her essay "Uses of the Erotic: The Erotic as Power" (1978), Audre Lorde puts forward a multifarious understanding of erotics that breaks with Freudian erotics by centralizing the racialized lesbian body and feminist antiracist struggle.[89] Audre Lorde was a poet, novelist, educator, and organizer, who carved out spaces of imagining the interlocking identities of being a black feminist, a lesbian, a mother, and a woman. On the one hand, Lorde was anything but asexual, as her journals, poetry, and biographer Alexis De Veaux speak to her relishing of sex, sexual love, and sexual seduction in her friendship groups and feminist circles.[90] Yet on the other hand, Lorde wrote and talked about erotics in a way that did not bind emotional depth and intimate relating to sex.[91] This is nowhere more clear than in her essay "Uses of the Erotic," which Lorde wrote four weeks before she found out she had breast cancer, in 1978, for the Fourth Berkshire Conference on the History of Women held at Mount Holyoke College.[92]

Writing against what she calls the "superficially erotic"—or what we might also think of as the codification of intimacy through the regime of sexuality—Lorde opens up space for a deep intimacy that is not reliant only on sex and sexuality for meaning but that finds satisfaction in a myriad of other activities and relationships to the self and to others.[93] Like with Freud, the erotic is an inner resource of power that fuels action and intimacy in the world. In distinction to Freud, however, Lorde's erotic is not a sexually motivated energy, instinct, or drive, making conceptual space for asexuality in a way that "sexuality" does not. If anything, it is the reverse: The erotic fuels sexual desire rather than sexual desire being at the base of the erotic. Sublimation, in this sense, drawing on a Lordean framework, is not the sublimation of sexual desires or a sexual drive into other life pursuits, but rather involves the transference of the erotic into various activities, sex included. This transformative understanding of the erotic, rather than sexual desire, as at the base of all creativity, marks Lorde's work as an intervention in Freudian-based understandings of the flows of desire and the well from which they spur.

While Lorde's essay relies on a strict gender binary that could be disadvantageous to imaging the gender dynamism of asexuality, I understand her grounding of the erotic in the "female plane" as speaking to a centralization of knowledge that has been epistemically discarded in patriarchal contexts through "male models of power" and a "racist, patriarchal, and anti-erotic society."[94] For instance, while Freud built psychoanalysis under a "male" principle that saw women as envious of masculinity (under the sign of the phallus) and thus wounded, Lorde envisions the erotic as a principle that white patriarchal society has ousted—reversing the terms of Freudian discourse and revaluing the feminine.[95] Reclaiming black lesbian feminist subjecthood as an epistemic standpoint from which the erotic generates thus means tapping into a "female" way of knowing and feeling—one that is distinct from sexual knowledge generation and its reliance on a god's-eye view and an assumed neutrality of white cisgender male subjecthood. Lorde's erotic aims to derive a different method and knowledge of the body and its actions in an unjust world. "The erotic is the nurturer or nursemaid of all our deepest knowledge," Lorde writes—a profound source of knowing *otherwise*.[96] In turn, the erotic is not obsessed with sexuality, sexual compartmentalization, or even sexuality's generation of identities from sexology henceforth. It is skeptical of the "european-american tradition, [where] need is satisfied by certain proscribed erotic comings-together" that restrict the erotic to "the bedroom alone."[97] In this sense, a Lordean erotic challenges the centralization of erotic activity under the act of "sex." A Lordean erotic is suspicious of sexuality as it exists in Western paradigms because it has marginalized and erased other forms of knowing and sensing while being "misnamed by men and used against women."[98] In these ways, Lorde mounts a challenge to sexology-derived and Freud-derived popularizations of the erotic that conflate it with sexuality.

Lorde articulates the erotic as expressed in several ways: through relationality or "sharing deeply any pursuit with another person," through allowing for joy and the knowledge of being capable of joy, through a knowledge of the self and a life lived with an attunement to an inner knowledge, and also with a commitment to refusing unjust deployments of erotics that make others tools of our own pleasure.[99] A Lordean erotic sees erotics and a critique of injustice as interconnected. To quote more extensively from Lorde, "the principal horror of any system which defines the good in terms of profit rather than in terms of human need, or which defines human need to the exclusion of the psychic and emotional components of that need—the principal horror of such a system is that it robs our work of its erotic value, its erotic power and life appeal."[100] In this way, the erotic is suggestive of a life energy of refusal and revolt, a critique of systems of oppression that strive to make one's labor, love, or time utilizable for the gain of others, thereby sapping one's erotic life energies. In this sense as well, the erotic becomes about more than fighting erotic injustice, drawing on Gayle Rubin's phrasing, it is also about developing erotic agency—the power to define, redefine, name, and assert in the face of social and discursive structures that encourage us to get in line, to tread a path, to be straightened into cooperation.[101] Yet a Lordean erotic is also about the mundane, and the erotic thrill of doing things for the self and others, deeply and with purpose, whether they be "dancing, building a bookcase, writing a poem, examining an idea."[102] It is through this variety of activities as meaningful that another asexual erotic is opened—attesting to the ways in which sex can be deemphasized as the most deep, meaningful, or erotic activity out there. What would it mean if social understandings of sexuality saw these actions—dancing, building a bookcase, writing a poem, examining an idea—as erotic, rather than affixing erotics to sex?[103] One answer to this lies with Awkward-Rich's opening to this book: Sex would be dismantled as the prima facie experience of love, bodily pride, and self-affirmation. This is the vision of this book as well as the vision of asexual erotics.[104]

A Lordean erotic unlocks an attention to both the mundane and the revolutionary, at once relational and rooted in self-empowerment on feminist terms. It envisions the erotic as beyond the sexual, evocative of life energies and deep seated emotional and psychic needs that cannot be enfolded within sexuality. It presents us with a distinct model for thinking about bodily knowledge and, as such, an alternative to sexual identity models. Erotics thus help to hone a distinction between sexuality as we know it and sexuality on different and other terms. Drawing on Lorde, the erotic opens up another mode of knowing and of acquiring knowledge and perhaps even another starting point for thinking a/sexual histories. Peter Coviello, in *Tomorrow's Parties: Sex and the Untimely in Nineteenth-Century America* (2013), contemplates modes of erotics in the nineteenth century that never ossified into recognizable sexual identities, lost possibilities that challenge the tautological progress narrative of sexual history and personal narratives of coming out.[105] Coviello, drawing on Michel Foucault's radical questioning of knowledge formation, undermines the assumption that past figures were unable to articulate gay, lesbian, bisexual, transgender, and asexual identities because they did not have the knowledge we contemporaries have at their disposal.[106] Instead, he suggests that sexual history is made because other erotic possibilities are unmade. In a similar way, Kathryn Kent explores romantic yet not necessarily sexual relatings between middle-class white women as queerly erotic in nature in ways that are not reducible to sexual identity and orientation.[107] Drawing on these insights, this book reflects on how asexual modes of relating have been set aside as compulsory sexuality and the centrality of sexual desire to modern subject formation has unfolded.

Crucially, the language of erotics also presents a response to theories that have tended, as Sharon Holland elucidates in *The Erotic Life of Racism* (2012), to separate sexuality from other aspects of social life and to establish sexuality as its own separate domain.[108] For instance, Tracy Bear discusses erotics in terms of "the sensualities of . . . body, mind, and spirit reunite[d]" and thus fundamental to all parts of life and living.[109] An attentiveness to erotics, following Holland and Bear, might thus also include disagreeing with Rubin's thesis that sexuality needs its own field of knowledge as a means to address erotic injustice.[110] What if the cordoning off of sexuality studies as a discreet, if interdisciplinary, field of knowledge has failed to attend fully to both the complexity of erotic injustice as well as to the ways in which erotics circulate on registers that are not and never were reducible to sexuality?

Multiple other theorists in recent years have drawn on Lorde to think about erotics in distinction or in addition to thinking sexuality—further pointing to the meanings this term carries for feminist thinking on relating. I want to review some of this work here because it provides further insight on how erotics can be utilized as a concept. "Erotics" appears centrally in Indigenous feminist and queer writing on sexuality and gender as a word that can be utilized to challenge the settler colonization of Indigenous sexualities and bodies by settler paradigms. Asserting erotic histories and presents of Indigenous people in contexts of settler colonialism, "Sovereign Erotics" emerge as Qwo-Li Driskill's term for "speaking of an erotic wholeness healed and/ or healing from the historical trauma that First Nations people continue to survive, rooted within the histories, traditions, and resistance struggles of our nations."[111] Similarly, Tracy Bear hones an "eroticanalysis" to explore "Indigenous erotics" and self-determination including through art, literature, and representation.[112] A Sovereign Erotics and Indigenous erotics work against the ways Indigenous people have been colonized while regrounding erotics in connection to "nations, traditions, and histories."[113] This is an approach that, like Lorde's, sees erotics in multiple facets of life rather than limited to sex and that grounds erotics in relations. As Mark Rifkin writes, "the erotic . . . speaks to a sense of embodied and emotional wholeness that includes but extends beyond the scenes and practices of sexual pleasure and gratification usually termed sexual."[114] Through focusing on erotics with Sovereign Erotics and Indigenous erotics, these texts invoke ways in which the erotic might be a term more amenable to projects of thinking intimate relating in excess of a regimented system of colonial sexuality.

In response to systems that harness our eroticism for the benefit of others, Mireille Miller-Young, writing on black women's agency in pornography, also puts forward "erotic sovereignty" as "a process . . . wherein sexual subjects aspire and move toward self-rule and collective affiliation and intimacy, and against the territorializing power of the disciplining state and social corpus."[115] In this sense, erotics can be utilized toward both critiquing injustice and reimagining agency on less restrictive terms. Finally, Angela Willey's explorations of monogamy have also drawn on Lorde's theorizations of erotics as distinct from sexuality. Like me, Willey sees in the erotic the possibility for thinking beyond sexual paradigms as they have been formulated. Further, the erotic for Willey opens up opportunities for critiquing sexuality itself. In her own words, "we must be willing to critique sexuality as we know it in order to understand . . . the erotic body. If we understand ourselves as 'erotic,' rather than (self-evidently, or universally) 'sexual,' our creaturliness has a different valence."[116] The erotic comes to stand in here as a wanting that cannot be encompassed by the sexual regime, the apparatus of sexuality wherein sex is prescribed as the remedy and sexual attraction is understood as the benchmark for desire and wanting.

While this book actively draws on the language of the erotic above and beyond that of sexuality as a concept that, as I have been arguing, creates possibilities for different ways of conceptualizing intimacy and relating, this is not to suggest that the erotic can be a space free of power. L. H. Stallings argues that all Eurocentric renderings of erotics and eros are caught up in truth systems around sexuality and based in white denials of the imaginative aspects of sexuality.[117] Further, Stallings's work calls into question the validity of seeking a transcendental erotics "as a concept that can be universally applied to various communities."[118] Thinking with these critiques, an emphasis on the erotic is thus only an attempt to think sexuality beyond sexual and bodily regimentation, an attempt to think through the well-known fact that there are many ways to love and be loved, to touch and be touched, to desire and be desired, to attract and be attracted, to arouse and be aroused that are not reducible to sex or encompassable by sexuality.

"Asexual erotics," drawing on this rich assemblage of writing but especially on Lorde's formulation, is a phrase I use to think about the critiques, forms of reading, and modes of relating that are made possible when asexuality is centralized. Much like heterosexuality is presumed to be the default for our socially enfleshed lives, so too *the sexual*—by which I mean being drawn to sex through sexual attraction and desire—is presumed to be our default orientation. This book in turn asks, how can we rethink relating when we read it asexually, rather than with an investment in the promises of sex and in the sexual universal?

I do this through a method of "asexual resonances" that involves undertaking an asexual reading of texts that may not be obviously asexual or that may not be identifiable as "asexual" in terms of orientatory definitions. This method assumes that "where there is queerness there is also asexuality," arguing that our investment in excavating queer genealogies, in particular, through an attachment to the sexual, has led to a tradition of neglect when it comes to asexuality.[119] This asexual reading practice involves remaining critical of how sex and sexuality are mobilized and toward what ends with the goal of interrogating compulsory sexuality. I understand the work of asexual critique and asexual identity as linked in the sense that asexual identity has made possible a critique of compulsory sexuality and desexualization. In turn, the work of critique can open up queer and feminist theoretical spaces to nonsexual and asexual contributions.

Many of the texts I examine are, in part, visual in nature; they are films and photographs. In analyzing these through a model of asexual resonances, I try to question and complicate what are perceived to be sexual motivations for relating—that is, the assumption that it is a desire for sex and sexual attraction that motivates people to form intimate bonds with one another. I have found that looking at how feminist, queer, and lesbian relating is represented in visual mediums is a potent strategy for asking what makes being drawn to another sexual, rather than, say, asexual. I suggest throughout that the motivation for relating—and especially feminist, queer, and lesbian relating—is not always sexual and often asexual in its erotics. This Lordean claim seems both obvious and overstated and yet little work has been done on exploring these asexual nodes of intimacy and what they might mean for understanding systems of sexuality.

*The erotic* is integral here because it assists me in thinking about relationality in a way that focusing on identity does not. While it is true that sexual identities are formed through relating to others (by way of "attraction"), this schema makes little sense for asexuality where attraction is not primarily sexual. The erotic, and especially a Lordean erotic, is thus a source of energy for thinking about how asexuality can be a sexual identity and orientation even while it can also be an affective, relational, and theoretical mode. Asexual erotics refer simultaneously to the erotics of asexual identity as to the "asexual" currents, moments, and erotic energies in all lives. Again, this practice is grounded in asexuality—and my own gray-asexuality, if you will—because it is only through asexuality that a sufficient critique of compulsory sexuality as limiting to people across spectrums and different positionalities can be developed.

Asexual erotics are suggestive of language that does not yet exist, of forms of erotic expression that are not feasible as identities or even nameable as properties in the first place. Asexuality and asexual erotic modes have figured as "nondiacritical differences," drawing again on Sedgwick's crucial insight that we tend to fixate on the gender of object choice in how we describe our erotic capacities, rather than on any number of other things.[120] Yet through the production of asexual identity, new and further "nondiacritical differences" are formed. Drawing again on Coviello's fascinating account of erotic expressions in nineteenth-century American writing, certain erotic expressions became unarticulateable with the crystallization of heterosexual and homosexual identities throughout the twentieth century. Coviello catalogues these erotic glimpses, asking, "What could have counted *as* sexuality? Was it a circumscribed set of bodily practices? A form of identification? A mode of relation? Was sexuality an aspect of one's identity?"[121] Drawing on Lorde, could it have been "dancing, building a bookcase, writing a poem, examining an idea"?[122] Or, drawing on Awkward-Rich, perhaps "Reading. Lying flat on [one's] back staring at the ceiling. Peeling back the skin of a grapefruit"?[123] Drawing on the erotic, I believe, allows for asexuality to be theorized on relational rather than singularly identitarian terms.

Further, exploring erotics on more expansive terms, which make space for asexual relating, is uniquely pertinent to contexts in which sexuality is compulsory and asexuality arises as an identifiable and nameable sexual identity. It is fascinating to think that the domain of sexuality is so codified that asexual modes of relating can be identifiable as a sexual identity in itself. In this sense, asexuality partakes in the "language [that] *solidif[ies]* . . . the very positing of something called sexuality as the self's most anxiously managed and tended-to property, something each of us is understood to *have*."[124] Throughout this book, in thinking about erotics rather than identification, I am interested in the ways that asexual flows are central to feminist, queer, and lesbian relating even while they often become understood on sexual terms. In thinking of an asexual erotics, this book is interested in challenging compulsory sexuality while drawing out erotic moments that also skirt around, radically refuse, or are adjacent to sexual expression.

## INTIMATE READINGS

In *Asexual Erotics* I get intimate with asexuality by reading compulsory sexuality through various modes of asexual erotics and their implications for feminist, queer, and lesbian theory, politics, representation, and relating. My chapters take up the temporal frame of the late 1960s onward, looking to feminist political celibacy/asexuality, lesbian bed death, the asexual queer child, and the aging spinster as four figures that are asexually resonant and that benefit from an asexual reading, from being read in an asexually affirming rather than asexually skeptical manner. While many late nineteenth- and early twentieth-century feminists were centrally invested in a politics of asexuality and spinsterhood that disrupted ties with men under patriarchy, this period lies outside of my temporal framework.[125] I begin with the late 1960s as a time when compulsory sexuality intensified and became increasingly tied, over subsequent decades, to feminist and later lesbian and queer notions of empowerment, politics, and subjectivity. Each chapter has something to say about asexual erotics, about the ways in which erotics have had asexual moments in feminist, lesbian, and queer countercultures. The chapters find it impossible and undesirable to separate the three domains of queer, feminist, lesbian from each other, just as I argue it is impossible to separate them from asexuality. The discursive, relational, and representational fields of feminist, queer, lesbian, and as I argue, asexual identities and politics are inextricably knotted with each other—they are co-constituting terms. What my analysis hopes to prove is not only that feminist, lesbian, queer are tangled terrains but also that they are erotically entangled with asexuality in ways that have gone unheeded.

Throughout *Asexual Erotics* I will use "nonsexuality" in addition to "asexuality."[126] While understanding the terms as related and overlapping, I think that "nonsexuality" is often a less contentious term and one that is not always identitarian in nature. "Asexuality," on the other hand, I put to use to ride the edge of asexual identification and the importance of arguing for its legitimacy as a sexual identity as well as the more relational, broader, more capacious, and less identitarian implications of the term. "Nonsexuality" is also a useful term because it helps make sense of the ways that various articulations and iterations of low sexual desire and sexual absence, although they have always existed, have not always been nameable as "asexuality" or coalesced under an identity of asexuality that has subjective meaning for those who use it.[127] Following on the work of Foucault and other historians of sexuality, it is possible to argue that "asexuality" has arisen as a sexual identity only within recent decades, as outlined earlier in the introduction.[128] While the book explores several forms of asexuality—political celibacy, lesbian bed death, intergenerational love, and aging adult spinsterhood—this list of asexual erotics could be extended to platonic love, Boston marriages, first-wave feminist chaste erotics, aphansis, so-called sexual desire disorders, frigidity, the figures of the prude and virgin, and religiously situated chastity.[129] Each has compelling asexual tales to tell that will require further rethinkings of sex, sexuality, feminism, queerness, lesbianism, and asexuality.

Notably, there have been several academic and popular books focused on various forms of nonsexualities in recent years, demonstrating the rising importance of this topic. For instance, queer theorist Michael Cobb has published *Single: Arguments for the Uncoupled* (2012), historians Alison Moore and Peter Cryle coauthored *Frigidity: An Intellectual History* (2011), and literary and queer theorist Benjamin Kahan has authored *Celibacies: American Modernism and Sexual Life* (2013). Also, popular books such as Rachel Hills's *The Sex Myth* (2015) and Kate Bolick's *Spinster: Making a Life of One's Own* (2015) likewise provide asexually resonant, and sometimes asexually explicit readings of popular culture.[130] Asexual, celibate, and nonsexual archives— much like gay, lesbian, bisexual, transgender, and queer ones—necessitate a broad understanding of identity, an eclecticism of cultural texts, and a feeling-based attunement in selecting these texts. This calls for "intimate readings" of compulsory sexuality—readings that are invested, asexually driven, and often autobiographically inflected. In undertaking my intimate readings, I rely on a feeling-based approach that examines sexuality through asexuality "haunted by the persistence of affect . . . across time."[131]

The story of *Asexual Erotics* begins with the women's liberation movement in the late 1960s and early 1970s. In "The Erotics of Feminist Revolution: Political Celibacies/Asexualities in the Women's Movement," I look at erotics as an energizing form of movement organizing rooted in challenging sexism, racism, classism, heteronormativity, and homophobia. Political celibacies/asexualities emerge here as an erotic component and central feminist tool of challenging injustice during that time period. I explore the theoretical and practical antiracist celibacy of Toni Cade Bambara and the Young Lords Party, the nihilist asexuality of Valerie Solanas, the separatist asexuality/celibacy of groups such as Cell 16 and The Feminists, and the lesbian celibacy of The Furies. I argue that feminism from the early moments of organizing has had strong *asexual* rather than sexual undercurrents that formed the ground for a particular erotics of the movement that has gone unexplored. I argue, more implicitly, that political celibacy/asexuality's dismissal from feminist accounts is drawn from the same fabric as widespread dismissal of asexual identity—namely, a system of compulsory sexuality that holds sex as central to relationality and community making while rendering asexuality, political celibacy/asexuality, and other nonsexualities backwards and "antisex." "The Erotics of Feminist Revolution" thus questions the categorical separation of celibacy from asexuality—that is, the separation of political identity and orientatory identity—arguing that both asexual modes exist in contexts of compulsory sexuality in which to be nonsexual is to be incomplete.

In the second chapter, "Lesbian Bed Death, Asexually: An Erotics of Failure," my object of study is lesbian bed death. Looking at the emergence of the concept of lesbian bed death as well as its presence in mainstream film and TV representations of lesbianism and lesbian art, I ponder on the erotics of what is perceived to be failed sexuality and the failure of lesbian identity. Providing an analysis of academic representations of lesbian bed death, I next explore how lesbian bed death is represented within popular representations of lesbians in television and film, and particularly in *The Fosters* (2013–2018) and *The Kids Are All Right* (2010). I argue that lesbian bed death's appearance and disappearance in these texts speaks to anxieties over lesbian identity and the role of sex within coalescing this identity. Asexuality, I suggest, comes to stand in as failed lesbianism even while it underwrites many moments within lesbian theorizing, including Boston marriages, intimate friendships, the woman-identified-woman of lesbian feminism, and lesbian and queer trauma. Next, I explore the figure of the bed in "lesbian art," such as in Tammy Rae Carland's *Lesbian Beds* series (2002) and Kyle Lasky's *Lesbian Bedrooms II* (2011), situating these visual representations of the bed as a politicized engagement that is resonant with asexuality. Throughout the chapter, I explore the erotic charge of asexuality for lesbianism as related to ideas of it as failure and in distinction to the happy poster child that asexuality is often required to be to gain credibility as a sexual identity in the first place. I identify this as, following Berlant and Edelman, an "asexuality without optimism," an erotics of failure which challenges celebratory identity politics.[132] Studying the "failure" of lesbian bed death, the chapter asks us to trouble happiness and wellness-centered narratives of asexuality, looking instead at the moribund registers of asexuality and how they do damage to capitalist ideals of productive selfhood.

The third chapter, "Growing into Asexuality: The Queer Erotics of Childhood," considers intergenerational erotics toward formulating a "growing into" rather than "growing out of" asexuality. While asexuality is commonly framed as a "phase" that one grows out of as one matures and approaches queer identity, I put forward that asexuality can be fruitfully understood as a "growing into." Beginning with an autobiographical remembering of intergenerational erotics, I explore both how childhood is desexualized and queer rebuttals of this desexualization. Following this, I turn to Maggie Nelson's "auto-theoretical" tribute to queer maternity and desire, *The Argonauts* (2015), reading the text from an asexually attuned perspective.[133] I argue that read alongside Valerie Solanas's *SCUM Manifesto, The Argonauts* offers us asexual intergenerational erotics founded on a "growing into" asexuality, queering and asexualizing stories of development. In the final portion of the chapter, I examine the work of two queer artists, Catherine Opie's *Self-Portrait/Nursing* (2004) and *Self-Portrait/Cutting* (1993) and Vivek Shraya's *Trisha* (2016), exploring how they further complicate our understandings of intergenerational sexuality through a "time spells" engagement with desire that challenges the typical temporalities of maturity narratives and intergenerational love.[134]

In the fourth chapter, "Erotics of Excess and the Aging Spinster," I contemplate the erotics of the aging spinster as an erotics of excess rather than lack and absence. Even while asexuality is held to be a site of sexual lack, thinking with the spinster I find that asexuality can also be understood as a site of erotic excess. Unpacking the desexualization of aging adults, the chapter provides a review of literature on sexuality and aging, arguing that it partakes in a misrendering of asexuality that has detrimental effects for both asexuality as an identity and older adults as a disenfranchised group. Turning toward the figure of the spinster in feminist work and examining the film *Frances Ha* (2012), directed by Noah Baumbach and written by Baumbach and Greta

Gerwig, I posit asexual erotics as an erotics of excess—in the sense of erotic excess, as an excess of whiteness, and as in excess of lesbian and heterosexual identity.[135]

Finally, in the epilogue, "Tyrannical Celibacy: The Anti-Erotics of Misogyny and White Supremacy," I turn to a recent series of events that took place in Toronto, Ontario, as I was finishing work on this book: a mass murder of pedestrians on a busy street corner that was done as a terrorist revenge crime by someone identified as an "incel"—an involuntary celibate. I explore how the existence of a misogynistic form of violence in the name of, or rather as a compensation for, "involuntary celibacy" functions as an expression of white entitlement that speaks to the importance of studying compulsory sexuality's entanglement with whiteness and patriarchy. Briefly looking at the history of the term "incel" and its uses, I demonstrate how feminist concepts including "injustice" and "celibacy" can ultimately be picked up in unpredictable ways. I argue that while similar in name to feminist political celibacy, involuntary celibacy, when practiced in tyrannical ways, is a form of anti-erotics that functions to quash the erotic expression of others as well as feminist and antiracist world transformation.

Taken together, *Asexual Erotics: Intimate Readings of Compulsory Sexuality* studies modern attachments to sex and sexuality and their constitutive role in feminist, lesbian, and queer scholarship. It explores attachments to the promises of sex through asexual resonances including the figures of political celibacy/asexuality, lesbian bed death, the queer asexual child, and the aging spinster, arguing for an asexual erotics that can stand as a queer feminist asexual articulation of relationality. In looking at filmic, fictional, online, photographic, and theoretical sources, *Asexual Erotics* assembles a compendium of asexual possibilities that speaks against the centralization of sex and sexuality within intimate subject formation and the dangerously unjust applications of compulsory sexuality.

CHAPTER 1

# The Erotics of Feminist Revolution

## Political Celibacies/Asexualities in the Women's Movement

IN A POSTER circulated in 1970s feminist communities, a pair of women lie entwined in bedcovers under a poster that reads "LESBIANS UNITE!" The photograph, captured by Donna Gottschalk in Pennsylvania, and printed by Times Change Press in 1971, proudly indicates that "SISTERHOOD FEELS GOOD" (see figure 1.1).[1] While it is difficult not to read the poster from today's vantage point as a celebration of a sexual lesbianism, or a celebration of lesbian sex, "SISTERHOOD FEELS GOOD" is evocative of a moment in lesbian feminism that was not strictly sexual—that is, a moment resonant with an asexual politics and erotics. As coeditor of the 1970s lesbian periodical *DYKE: A Quarterly of Lesbian Culture and Analysis* and former owner of one of the posters, Liza Cowan, indicates: "The fact that the women are in bed, but in bed sleeping said everything good to me. Today, the image would be all about sex [and] . . . that wasn't the only, or, for me, the main point."[2] The poster instead signified an aspirational sisterhood that was grounded in an antiracist, antisexist, and antihomophobic erotics—an erotics of organizing for revolution.

When I was teaching one of the first university courses ever offered on asexuality worldwide in the fall of 2017, the students explored concepts of the erotic, drawing especially on Audre Lorde.[3] In one class, when discussing what we each found erotic in our own lives and experiences, one student confessed that she finds political organizing erotic.[4] Her use of "erotic" here, grounded in the reading we did of Lorde, is not to be understood as

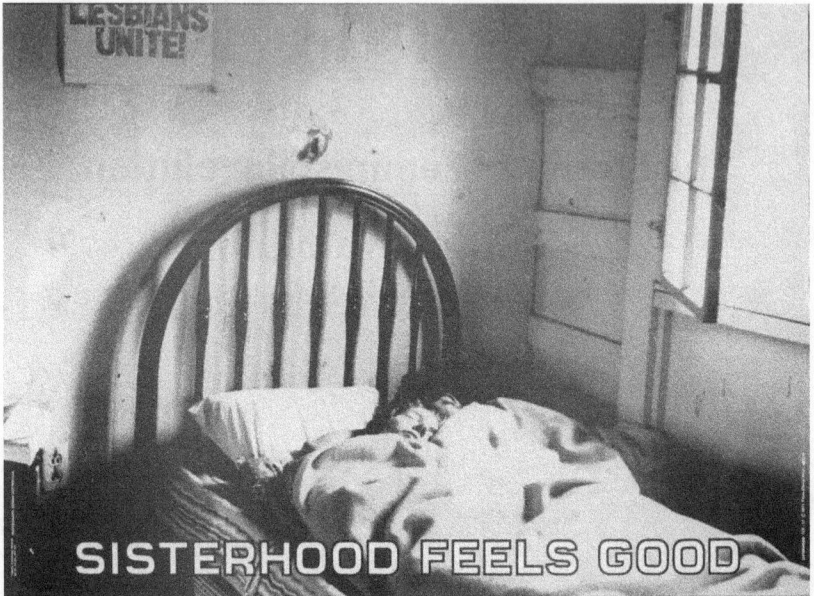

**FIGURE 1.1.** "SISTERHOOD FEELS GOOD," printed as an offset lithograph by Times Change Press circa 1971, with photograph by Donna Gottschalk, 1969. Reprinted with the permission of Donna Gottschalk. Image provided by the Oakland Museum of California, with thanks to Brittany Bradley, Intellectual Property and Imaging Coordinator.

reducible to sexual energy but rather refers to the energies of collaboration, solidarity, and antiracist feminist organizing. In ways that echo this student's statement, the erotic, drawing on Lorde, proved in the 1960s and 1970s to be a formidable resource that allowed organizers, activists, and writers to challenge injustice. Lorde argued that women are encouraged to separate the erotic from vital aspects of life and channel it solely into sex because when erotic energies are channeled away from sex and toward life making or revolution, women become "dangerous."[5] In turn, through "recognizing the power of the erotic" feminists "pursue[d] genuine change within [their] world[s] . . . in the face of a racist, patriarchal, and anti-erotic society."[6] This utilization of the erotic was grounded in collective struggle against injustice, "deep participation" as Lorde calls it, which made the fight against injustice possible in the first place.[7] Drawing on this ideation of erotics as not only bound to sexual desire but rooted in an intimate challenging of sexism, racism, classism, and homophobia opens up space for political celibacies/asexualities to be formulated as erotic rather than as against erotics, as they have often been framed under monikers of "sex negativity." This chapter considers erotics in seeking to tell the story of a particularly vital and complex moment in feminist history through an asexually attuned reading.

My discussion in this chapter looks at the erotic valence of political asexuality/celibacy in feminist communities of the women's liberation movement. While there are clearly asexual politics intrinsic to earlier feminist movements, including first-wave feminisms, as evidenced by appeals to chastity in an age prior to widespread access to birth control technologies, I focus on the asexual politics arising in the North American, and primarily US context of the women's liberation movement of the sixties and seventies on. Reading feminist periodicals from the late sixties, seventies, and even eighties, I find it surprising just how often a politics of celibacy and asexuality comes through. *No More Fun and Games,* and many other feminist journals, including *Off Our Backs, The Lesbian Feminist, Sinister Wisdom, Dyke, TRIBAD: Lesbian Separatist Journal, Lesbian Connection, The Tide,* and then in the eighties *Heresis* and *The Celibate Woman,* published a variety of pieces on political celibacy/asexuality. Political feminist celibacy/asexuality came to constitute an active politics, praxis, and theory for feminists to revoke their emotional, reproductive, and labor-intensive support from men and instead direct it to themselves, other women, and movement struggles. Alongside agitating for access to abortion, contraception, rape prevention, and freedom from sterilization, fighting racism and homophobia, mapping women's pleasures such as through the embracing of the clitoris, and the articulation of lesbianism as a practice of feminism, political celibacy and political asexuality arose as a competent feminist strategy for theorizing and practicing feminist bodily autonomy and ulterior community formation. Notably, the terms "asexuality" and "celibacy" were used more or less interchangeably, both denoting a political and erotic distancing from sex.[8] This is significant because it marks the two terms as equally politicized and indicative of a tactical disengagement from sex. As I discuss later in this chapter, while "sex" was in the first instance understood on heterosexual terms, this asexual energy also animated early lesbian feminist organizing.

The late 1960s and early 1970s offer a historical moment when asexuality and celibacy were widely theorized and mobilized in the face of sexism and racism as feminist tactics among black and antiracist feminists as well as within white feminist circles. Black and antiracist feminists grounded in multiple movement struggles, including Black Power, developed distinct articulations of celibacy that were aimed at challenging sexism toward developing group and individual wholeness and combating a racist society. For example, writer and public intellectual Toni Cade Bambara theorized political celibacy as a way to build wholeness, increase self-autonomy, and address sexism and racism simultaneously.[9] The women in the Puerto Rican antiracist group the Young Lords Party, on the other hand, undertook a sex strike so as to force increased attention on male machismo within the group, and thereby build a stronger base from which to challenge racism.[10] Within a less racism-aware framework, political asexuality/celibacy took off in feminist separatist and radical communities after the uptake of Valerie Solanas's *SCUM Manifesto*, published following her shooting of artist Andy Warhol in 1968.[11] In *SCUM*, Solanas polemically proposes a nihilistic asexuality that would both unfasten women from their labor as biological reproducers of children and bring on the demise of patriarchy. The *SCUM Manifesto* became commonly read and influential in the formation of separatist feminist organizing, including among the two groups The Feminists and the Boston women's group Cell 16, which published the periodical *No More Fun and Games* (1968–1973). Also, a particular stream of celibacy emerged within lesbian feminist communities such as The Furies, in Washington, DC. As a strain of feminist thought, and one linked strongly with separatism, lesbianism, and antiracist organizing, political celibacy/asexuality was both tactical and ideological, creating ground for bringing women together and providing creative tools for survival in contexts of impeded bodily autonomy. Interestingly, even while political celibacy/asexuality fell sharply out of favor in North America in the late 1980s, 1990s, and the first decade of the 2000s and became understood in terms of "sex negativity," feminist and women's groups in multiple locations around the world (including Ukraine, Liberia, Japan, and Columbia) have since enacted "sex strikes" in pursuit of peace and justice, suggesting its widespread importance as a feminist revolutionary tactic.

While the work of Solanas and members of radical, separatist, and lesbian feminist communities is often framed as solely trans-exclusionary, several scholars have argued that trans women were part of radical and lesbian feminist communities and that some groups were invested in trans-inclusionary practices that sought to protect trans women from vitriol. Cristan Williams and Finn Enke detail the ways, for example, in which Olivia Records, which was a separatist lesbian feminist music collective influential in the 1970s and born from The Furies, came together to protect sound engineer Sandy Stone from attacks on the veracity of her womanness by trans-exclusionary feminists.[12] Even while grounded in commitments to separatism, the feminist separatism of the late sixties and early seventies was not always (though importantly, it was at other times) invested in excluding transgender women. For instance, Ti-Grace Atkinson, who founded the group The Feminists, has in the last decade come to prominence for espousing persistently trans-exclusionary rhetoric, while her contemporaries Dana Densmore and Roxanne Dunbar-Ortiz of the former feminist separatist group Cell 16 have refused to get on board.[13] Further, the writings and groups that enacted and theorized political asexuality/celibacy, as I will explore, were often grounded in biological determinism and the gender binary, though they also often undercut their own assertions of biological certainty. While I do not think that political celibacy/asexuality is inherently trans-exclusionary, the groups I examine consisted, with one exception and to the best of my knowledge, of only cisgender women (as well as, though not described on these terms, masculine of center, gender-variant, and perhaps nonbinary individuals).[14]

This chapter proceeds with a consideration of the relationship between political celibacy/asexuality and the contemporary sexual orientation of asexuality, arguing for the relevancy of one for the other. Next, I examine the erotic context of the sixties and seventies, arguing that while these decades (and the sixties in particular) are often framed as about "free love" and "sexual liberation," these framings miss the point of the way erotics circulated in the manifold revolutions that were taking place at the time as well as of the deeply seated sexism and racism that made sexual availability often oppressive rather than liberating for women. Following on this, I explore several compelling instances of erotic political celibacies/asexualities of the sixties and seventies: antiracist celibacies, nihilist asexuality, separatist celibacies, and lesbian celibacies. While these categories are not intended to be definitive, they provide a sense of the many uses that feminists of the sixties and seventies found for political celibacy/asexuality. I examine the politics of antiracist, nihilist, separatist, and lesbian celibacies each in turn with attention to how political asexuality/celibacy was articulated and how it was leveraged against oppressive systems either theoretically or in application. I argue that political celibacy/asexuality was a central axis and erotic setting within feminist thought and practice in the late sixties and seventies and one that constituted a challenge to sexism, racism, classism, heteronormativity, and homophobia.

## ASEXUAL ORIENTATION AND POLITICAL CELIBACY/ASEXUALITY: WHAT IS AT STAKE?

Feminist scholar Breanne Fahs, in "Radical Refusals: On the Anarchist Politics of Women Choosing Asexuality" (2010), has argued that while ignored in contemporary and recent feminist sexuality studies, political celibacy/asexuality is a compelling "radical refusal," an anarchist and feminist strategy against a type of sex that constrained women while binding them to men.[15] Fahs asks evocatively, "What if women *stopped* having sex permanently?"—suggesting in response to her own question that it would constitute an undercutting of patriarchal institutions such as the family and of gendered power dynamics.[16]

Yet Fahs's work has not been warmly received by asexual communities, on account that it partakes in a collapse of the differences between particular historical contexts (namely, the late 1960s and early 1970s, on the one hand, and the first decade of the 2000s, on the other), and even more so of *political* asexuality and asexual *identity* and *orientation*.[17] For instance, asexual activists have argued that Fahs does a disservice to the sexual orientation and identity of asexuality, because she does not draw out the differences between asexual identity and feminist asexual politics, suggesting that asexuality is, point factum, a political orientation, rather than an inherently sexual orientation like any other. In other words, the sentiment of asexual activists is such that for asexuality to gain credibility as a sexual orientation, it is damaging to portray it as a politically motivated choice.

At the same time, the direction of feminist and queer work on asexuality in recent years, as outlined in the introduction, has begun to create possibilities for asexuality as both a sexual identity and a base from which to investigate feminist commitments to sex. It thus seems possible to honor the sexual identity and orientation of asexuality, and the experiences of people across the asexuality spectrum, while also studying the feminist celibacies or asexualities of the women's movement and beyond. This chapter undertakes a retrieval of political celibacy/asexuality that stems from an asexually motivated reading, and that sees asexual identity and political celibacy/asexuality as related, cousined, and allied—if also distinct—terms and iterations of nonsexuality. More to the point, I want to argue that discriminatory and marginalizing intentions toward asexuality stem from the very same fountain as feminist inattentiveness to political celibacy/asexuality. If the routine disbelief and disqualification of asexuality as a legitimate sexual identification spurs from the belief that sex and sexual desire are central organizing forces for all modern subjects, then the concomitant absenting of political feminist celibacy/asexuality as well as its framing as a threat to contemporary sex-positive feminism stems from a feminist conviction or feeling that sex and sexual desire are central to all feminist subjects.

In other words, both feminist theory's reluctant approach to political celibacy/asexuality and broader social hesitancy to recognize asexuality as a sexual orientation are informed by what critical disability and asexuality studies scholar Eunjung Kim has identified as an "asexphobia."[18] Asexuality, as discussed in the introduction, is often perceived as a disorder, a phase, a sign of immaturity or lack of self-knowledge, and—in the case of feminist and queer communities—as a prudish, antisex threat to the very notion of feminism and queerness as well as to the fabric of the feminist and queer community. As asexuality studies scholars KJ Cerankowski and M. Milks point out, asexuality "challeng[es] many of the basic tenets of pro-sex feminism," asking us to rethink the pitting of transgressive sexualities against "anti-sex" sexualities.[19] Yet with asexuality gaining headway into queer and feminist politics, as evidenced by burgeoning literature and online activisms, I grow more and more convinced of the possibilities for an asexual criticism that questions feminist and queer attachments to sex. Working in this moment and drawing on its energy, I turn to the feminist politics of radical celibacy and asexuality in its multiple forms not only to add some descriptive thickness to a thread of feminism more or less forgotten but also as a means to ponder how it is that this mode of asexual corporeal engagement felt political and erotic.

## THE EROTIC SIXTIES AND SEVENTIES

Political celibacies and political asexualities, no less than other practices of alternate world making, constitute a queer challenge to heteronormative times, rhythms, institutions, relations, and power flows. As Victoria Hesford frames it, the second wave was about "taking the risk of becoming strange in relation to gender and sex norms," and in this sense, "it was something closer to what we now call 'queer'—a practice of subverting and living against, or across, social identities."[20] Through providing an alternate geometry of relating that deemphasized sex, fought for the end of "sex-based" and race-based inequalities in relation to hetero-patriarchy, imagined new ways of inhabiting life, and fostered the emergence of a sensual asexual erotics, political celibacies/asexualities can be read from today's vantage point as imbued with a certain queerness. In imagining a denial of sex, feminists undertook a radically queer approach to subverting both gendered norms and ideas and the structures that enabled them—including patriarchy, white supremacy, and heterosexuality.

Political celibacy/asexuality—indeed, political celibacies/asexualities in the plural—demonstrated a political engagement with the competing discourses of the era. The 1960s are historically remembered as a decade of revolutionary action and change within America: civil rights struggles to end racial apartheid in the South, the Black Power movement's assertion of black identity and struggle against socially sanctioned racism, the American Indian Movement's fight to draw attention to the genocidal intentions of settler colonialism, antiwar organizing in opposition to the Vietnam War, the

LGBT rights movement's fight against homophobia, and the women's liberation movement's stand against sex-based discrimination. These movements
were interconnected, rather than separated, and informed by shifting ideas
around sexuality and sex.

Jane Gerhard, in *Desiring Revolution* (2001), a history of sexuality and the
women's movement, argues that "there was a period in the late 1960s and early
1970s when sex mattered in a whole new way."[21] On the one hand, sexological
discourse such as the work of famed William Masters and Virginia Johnson
sought to establish women as equally sexually desiring, arousable, and orgasmic as men, arguing for the similarity between women's and men's sexualities,
the sameness of their sexual response cycles, and the functional similarity
between the clitoris and penis.[22] Against the backdrop of this research, a "per-
missive turn" began to flourish in America, a "shift toward a more libertarian
ethic [of sex]."[23] Whether "more rhetoric than reality," the so-called sexual revolution, bolstered by the appearance of the contraceptive pill in the sixties, saw
the marketing of sex and sexual lifestyles to white middle-class Americans,
as evinced most notably by Hugh Hefner's *Playboy,* first published in 1953,
and Helen Gurley Brown's *Sex and the Single Girl,* published in 1962, which
encouraged readers to like sex and discouraged any sign of "frigidity," while
avoiding discussion of abortion or contraception.[24] Challenging monogamy
but upholding heterosexuality, texts such as these spoke to a sexual liberaliza-
tion and an imagined equality between men's and women's engagement with
ideas of sexual freedom. In the words of feminist Ti-Grace Atkinson, because
sex-based discrimination and inequality persisted, and because "no birth control was fail-safe and yet everything pushed you to having sex," "women lost
not only the right to expect traditional forms of exchange for sex (love, commitment, marriage), but also the 'morally based' grounds on which to refuse
sex they did not want."[25] As feminist organizer active in Cell 16, Roxanne Dunbar-Ortiz wrote: "The confidence that sexuality is the source of human liberation must be questioned. . . . With all the talk of sexual liberation, one rarely
hears talk of the liberation from sexuality, which many women privately voice.
Such a sentiment reveals, so men say, 'frigidity,' 'coldness,' Brave New World
surrealism."[26] In other words, as sex became normalized for white women outside martial contexts, heterosexuality became further entrenched and frigidity
arose in prominence as a pathological trait used pejoratively against women
who were not sexually active with men.

At the same time, as sexual prowess was being extended to some women,
virginity and sexual restraint continued to be socially rewarded ideals for
many women. These competing sexist claims suggested that, on the one hand,
women *should* be sexually adventurous and sexually available for men under

the rubrics of free love, hippiedom, and 1960s liberality, even despite a persistent attachment to the virginal, presexual, or "asexual" ideal for women. Yet this "asexual ideal," asexuality studies scholar Ianna Hawkins Owen argues, has functioned historically as an ideal of white femininity, invested in white mastery, morality, and sexual restraint.[27] In the mid-1960s, the incredibly damaging Moynihan Report authored by Daniel Moynihan, titled *The Negro Family: The Case for National Action* (1965), was published, essentially blaming black women for poverty in black communities through the suggestion that powerful matriarchs were emasculating men.[28] Patricia Hill Collins demonstrates how the ideas put forward by the Moynihan Report supported constraining and pernicious ideas around black women's sexualities intent on exerting control over their reproductive freedom. "Controlling images" such as the desexualized "mammy," the "matriarch," the "welfare mother," and the "jezebel" emerged here as tools of a white supremacist patriarchy, "reflecting the dominant group's interest in maintaining Black women's subordination."[29] While the desexualized "mammy" provided a "safe" image of black femininity ever ready for exploitation in the white household, the "jezebel" figure was rendered as an oversexed and sexually aggressive woman, justifying her sexual exploitation by white men.[30] Further, while the "mammy" was the "good" figure of black maternity, the "matriarch" figure supported by the Moynihan Report and the "welfare mother" provided schemas for black feminine culpability and "bad" motherhood.[31] In all of these figurations, sexuality arose as a key terrain for black women's oppression and subjugation, demonstrating that so-called free love operated alongside persistent and ardent racism and sexism.

Puerto Rican, Native American, and black women were also routinely desexualized during the era through forced and coerced sterilization, so that while white women were fighting for access to safe abortion and contraception, women of color were frequently fighting against coerced sterilization.[32] In the 1960s, for instance, the development of the birth control pill utilized the bodies of Puerto Rican women as test subjects, and up to one third of Puerto Rican women were sterilized from the 1930s to the 1960s.[33] Native American women in the US and Indigenous women in Canada have likewise faced widespread and government- and corporation-funded coerced sterilization in the 1960s and 1970s.[34] In *The Black Woman,* one essay by Toni Cade Bambara asks, "The Pill: Genocide or Liberation?," seeing "the bomb, the gun, the pill" as similar tools of colonial violence—a stipulation that, as Margo Natalie Crawford points out, would not have made any sense to white feminists of the era.[35] Further, even while the 1960s are understood as a decade of "free love," Winifred Breines, in *The Trouble Between Us* (2006), demonstrates that civil rights organizing in the 1960s, as well as the liberal left, was thick with a "virtual panic and pathology around interracial sex," pointing to the limits of the sexual "liberation" of the era.[36]

Kimberly Springer argues that feminist organizing in 1960s and 1970s America developed, in large part, along racially segregated lines.[37] She lists four reasons why black women intentionally did not align themselves with the white women's liberation movement, including to solidify relations with black men and thus keep communities and the black movement intact and strong, to not divert energy away from the civil rights and black movements, because of a historically founded distrust between black women and white women, and because of racist histories and cultural stereotypes.[38] Disagreeing with this argument, the editors of *Want to Start a Revolution?* (2009) demonstrate that black women were deeply embedded in—rather than external to—both black freedom and feminist struggles of the era.[39] Similarly, Sherie Randolph argues that black feminists acted as bridge-builders between movements as well as creators of a black feminist movement. For example, she demonstrates that lawyer Florynce (Flo) Kennedy, active in the civil rights, Black Power, and feminist struggles, was a major, if often unacknowledged, architect of the women's liberation movement.[40]

The black women's movement had an intersectional and interlocking "black feminist consciousness" that elaborated the double, triple, or multiple jeopardy of race and gender and existed parallel to what became, in large part, a women's liberation movement invested in an uninterrogated whiteness.[41] Multiple organizations took form in the 1960s and 1970s aimed at central-izing the experiences of black women and women of color, such as the Third World Women's Alliance, formed in 1968, which authored *Triple Jeopardy*; the National Black Feminist Organization, founded in 1973 by Flo Kennedy; the black feminist lesbian organization Combahee River Collective, founded in 1974; and Women of All Red Nations, also founded in 1974. These groups responded to the lack of focus on racism in the women's movement and artic-ulated new visions for revolution.

Unlike many white feminists of the era, black feminists and feminists of color of the 1960s were not invested in examining "sex-based" oppression out-side of or apart from considerations of racism, colonialism, and class. As Toni Cade Bambara speaks to in the introduction to *The Black Woman* (1970)—a pivotal text in the shaping of 1970s black feminism—neither the perspectives of white feminists nor those of black male intellectuals and nationalists suf-ficed epistemically.[42] Faced with racism in many feminist communities, sexism in some black communities, and the intersections of these in day-to-day life, black feminists formulated complex accounts that interrogated both whiteness and heteropatriarchy. For example, as the Combahee River Collective State-ment famously indicates, they were "actively committed to struggling against racial, sexual, heterosexual, and class oppression, [through] the development of integrated analysis and practice based upon the fact that the major systems of oppression are interlocking."[43]

Claims of the sixties and seventies being a time of "sexual liberation" ulti-mately fail at conceptualizing the complexity of issues facing women in this era—drawing attention away from how sexuality was not by any means "free love" for women under conditions of continuing racism and sexism. Sex and freedom, as this chapter will continue to explore, were often formulated by feminists and women of this era as separate terrains rather than correlated ones. Indeed, the accounts of political celibacy/asexuality I examine often implicitly asked the question Hawkins Owen has raised: "Why have sex when you can have freedom?"[44] Indeed, many of the "freedom dreams" elaborated by feminists of the era—drawing on the language of historian Robin Kelley—were about seeking freedom *from* the oppression that was understood to be related to sex in contexts of sexism, racism, and heteropatriarchy.[45] A fram-ing of the sixties or seventies as about free love and sexual liberation also misses the intensity of political struggles taking place at the time, which, while entwined with sexuality, were not ever solely about access to sex, as demon-strated by the manifold accounts of political celibacy/asexuality that I will proceed to outline. I thus suggest instead that these were "erotic" decades fueled by multifarious erotics—as much about the erotic energies of political organizing as they were about the erotic energies of sexual revolution.

## ANTIRACIST CELIBACIES

Celibacy itself has functioned historically as a lily-white ideal of sexual restraint available mostly to white men and women. In white supremacist and sexist contexts throughout US history, women of color, including black women, have routinely faced sexual violence and forced sterilization, con-straining possibilities for celibate practices and identities. Kathryn Kent argues that in the postbellum period and the early twentieth century, marriage sig-nified differently for white women and black women such that white women sought self-autonomy through refusing marriage while black women sought self-determination and entry into the public sphere through marrying.[46] For example, in the early twentieth century, prominent African American intel-lectual and romantic novelist Pauline Hopkins advocated against "marriage resistance" for black women, arguing instead for "developing pleasant homes and beautiful families."[47] Hawkins Owen has also explored how celibacy has often been imposed on black women as a result of state intervention. When interviewing Black Panther party member Ericka Huggins, Hawkins Owen found that Huggins experienced imposed celibacy, or "a kind of stillness," during a fourteen-month period of incarceration.[48] As mentioned, the eugenics-grounded sterilization of women of color, including Puerto Rican, black, and Native American women, has likewise led to circumstances of imposed rather than self-chosen celibacy.

Similar arguments can also be made in terms of black masculinity. The hypersexualization of black men under white supremacy to justify the "protection" of white women's chasteness suggests, for example, that white women's "celibacy" has been a tool used to justify racist hatred. Further, the very terms of the Moynihan Report describe black men as "emasculated" or "castrated" by black matriarchs, terminology laden with an imposed celibacy not of one's own making.[49] These fears of forced, coerced, or imposed celibacy are likewise evident in black masculinist discourse of the era, which struggled for black masculine pride through, in part, asserting sexual access to women.[50] Imposed celibacy in the form of language of "emasculation," "castration," and "de-balling/deballing" appears in the sixties as a common metaphor for the oppression of black masculinity, attempts to silence black men, as well as fears of feminism and the "black matriarch," demonstrating the integral role of sexual prowess to radical black masculine identity as well as grounded fears of forced celibacy. For example, Gwen Patton, published in *The Black Woman* collection, writes that "black women have been cagey about their comments and contributions to the [Black Power] Movement for fear of de-balling the needed and well-loved new leaders," indicating that desexualization and imposed celibacy had toxic and inhibiting effects for both men and women in the Black Power movement.[51]

Yet, researching political celibacies in the sixties and seventies, I found several compelling articulations and practices of strategic political celibacy as an approach to striving toward antiracist and antisexist realities. This led me to ask whether and to what extent political asexuality/celibacy was formulated as part of an antiracist feminist position in the context of the sixties and seventies under continuing white supremacy, racial injustice, and the hypersexualization of black femininity. Further, how has political celibacy functioned differently for black women and women of color struggling against racism and sexism than it has for white women whose focus in the sixties and seventies was primarily on "sex-based" oppression?[52]

With several exceptions, little work has been undertaken exploring celibacy as a political tool that can theoretically and practically provide a resource for antiracist and feminist struggles. In *Celibacies,* Benjamin Kahan argues that forms of nonsexuality such as celibacy are a sexual identity and not simply a pre-gay identification or form of repression. In one chapter in particular, Kahan traces the celibate politics of black religious figure of the late Harlem Renaissance of the 1930s, Father Divine.[53] With a large following, Father Divine encouraged interracial communes as a strategy for navigating antiblack racism in the US—facilitating, for example, the purchase of land and property and resource pooling (Kahan calls this "celibate economics").[54] Most fascinatingly, as Kahan discusses, Father Divine espoused celibacy among his followers as a radical antiracist strategy. Through celibacy, Father Divine "counter[ed] dehumanizing depictions of black sexuality" as hypersexualized and effected material prosperity among many of his followers at a time when Theodore Roosevelt's New Deal was implemented after the Great Depression to protect the employment of white men over men of color (domestic and agricultural workers—large numbers of whom were African American—were not protected by the Social Security Act of 1935).[55] Further, through political celibacy, Father Divine encouraged the building of antiracist communal living in response to "the inadequacy of the nuclear family," meanwhile redefining the white contours of celibate practice.[56] I draw on Kahan's discussion of Father Divine because it provides a rare and vivid depiction of how celibacy, in the face of historical deployments of celibacy as a white politics of sexual restraint, has been utilized as a tool toward antiracist ends. I build on Kahan's work by examining the antiracist political celibacies articulated by Toni Cade Bambara and enacted by the Young Lords Party.

Writer, professor, activist, organizer, and screenplay writer Toni Cade Bambara in "On the Issue of Roles" (1969/1970), delivered as part of a lecture in 1969 and published in her groundbreaking volume *The Black Woman* (1970), offers a politicized antiracist conceptualization of celibacy.[57] Brittney Cooper writes that 1970 was an auspicious year for "Black women's cultural and intellectual intelligibility" and the start of a "veritable Black women's literary renaissance" with the publication of books by Alice Walker, Toni Morrison, Maya Angelou, and Ida B. Wells's posthumous autobiography.[58] *The Black Woman* was a first-of-its kind collection that included a variety of academic and activist perspectives that refused a singular articulation of blackness or womanhood and disrupted both an arising white feminist and black male intellectual canon.[59] In one of her own pieces in the volume, "On the Issue of Roles," Bambara develops a critique of compulsory sexuality and a suggestion of celibacy along two lines: self-autonomy and wholeness.[60] First, Bambara questions white capitalist gender roles and complicates the gender binary through asserting the need for, "above all, total self-autonomy."[61] When sex is used as a white supremacist tool, Bambara suggests, it antagonizes men and women and prevents both from achieving creative agency over their lives and effectively organizing for revolution. Because white models of gender have been inflicted through colonization, black communities, Bambara argues, have been formed along divisive, gendered lines that prevent both self-autonomy for men and women as well as wholeness for individuals and the community. Sex is implicated in this because it serves to support rather than undermine, in her view, the gender binary and the antagonistic relationship between men and women. Bambara thus writes that "celibacy for a time is worth considering, for sex is dirty if all it means is winning a man, conquering a woman, beating someone out of something, abusing each other's dignity in order to prove that I am a man, I am a woman."[62] This complex statement indicates a critique of compulsory sexuality and an insistence that sex is "dirty" in white colonial contexts because it is used as a tool of oppression and of enforcing subjugated gender status. The "dirtiness" of sex is its inherent tie to white supremacist models of relating through gendered antagonism and gender-based oppression. Whereas the Moynihan Report created the conditions for antagonistic relating between men and women as a means for "the oppressor . . . to create havoc and discord among the colonized," Bambara envisions celibacy as a potential salve for making the self and community whole and altering oppressive gender relations.[63] Because, as Bambara writes, "it doesn't take any particular expertise to observe that one of the most characteristic features of our community is the antagonism between our men and our women," celibacy is articulated as a way to dismantle the oppressive polarization of gendered norms in antiblack racist contexts.[64] Bambara argues against the fragile emasculated male—with, in her own words, "lost-ball fantasies"—working against constraining definitions of black masculinity and femininity.[65] Bambara thus presents strategic political celibacy as a potential tool in the antiracist feminist tool kit, one that can reshift relations between men and women and encourage black men and women to work toward dismantling a racist state and internalized racism. Political celibacy functions in this sense as a strategy for black women to seek self-autonomy, a strategy for black men to question the function of sexism in masculinity, and a strategy for seeking wholeness more broadly. In her own words, "revolution for self is all about—the whole person."[66]

The political erotics formulated here are nonsexual in the way that they harness episodic celibacy toward building deeper love, knowledge, wholeness, and anti-oppressive communities. Because "revolution begins with the self, in the self," celibacy fosters an altered relationship with one's own erotic energy and with one's capacity to be erotically invested with others in revolutionary struggle.[67] Political celibacy as geared toward an erotics of wholeness reso-nates, it might be added, with Lorde's formulation of erotics as a resource at once greater, broader, and deeper than sexuality and as geared toward auton-omy and wholeness. Lorde wrote of honing wholeness and autonomy within antiracist organizing, pointing out that sexism also diminishes black men and that women and men must come together as "self-actualized individuals."[68] As part of a distinct articulation of a black feminist epistemology for disrupting patterns of oppressively gendered relating imposed by white supremacy, Bam-bara directs our attention to ways in which political celibacy can be leveraged to theorize liberation grounded in anti-oppressive self-knowledge.

It is also worth noting that Bambara was not alone in formulating politi-cal celibacy as an antiracist tool of Black Power for shifting white patterns of gendered relating. Poet Bob Bennett in *Black Fire* (1968) offers a feminist anti-racist view on masculinity likewise invested in political celibacy.[69] In a poem named "(Title)," Bennett puts forward a vision for "nonromantic, nonsexual relations" between men and women.[70] Rather than drawing on the language of "emasculation" or imposed celibacy or on the "toxic" matriarchal house-hold as outlined in the Moynihan Report, Bennett imagines an ulterior model for family, love, and masculinity based on love between siblings—"sisters and brothers."[71] Bennett writes, "(She is my sister: I am her brother) / Without romance there is love," depicting a sisterly-brotherly erotics rooted in revo-lution rather than in what has been termed "amatonormativity," or the pres-sure to form romantic couples above and beyond other relational formations.[72] While filial bonds of "brotherhood" were key to Black Power, Bennett expands this to a sisterhood/brotherhood that is not attached to sex or romance. Here a self-chosen celibacy emerges as an aromantic relational mode invested with revolutionary erotics and the power to transform relating between women and men under white supremacist patriarchy. "Love" emerges as more pertinent than sex or even romance, as rooted in the revolutionary language of sister-hood and brotherhood, and as invested, as with Bambara, in seeking whole-ness in the self and in the community.

While Bambara and Bennett articulate forms of political celibacy on paper, the National Young Lords Party (YLP) undertook political celibacy in prac-tice as a tool toward ending sexism in an antiracist organization. The Young Lords Party was a Puerto Rican organization formed in 1969 and grounded in an anticolonial history and Puerto Rican nationalist struggles, with a broad membership that included many African Americans and non–Puerto Rican Latinx bonded through radical struggle (around 30 percent of its members were not Puerto Rican).[73] Based first in Chicago, the group quickly expanded to New York (East Harlem and South Bronx). Alongside reading theory, they published the bilingual newspaper *Pa'lante* (also written as *Palante*), which offered antiracist coverage on local and international struggles, and undertook activist interventions in communities, such as garbage dumping to enforce the pickup of garbage by the city of New York, anti–lead poisoning organizing, and other forms of health activism.[74] The Young Lords Party demanded Puerto Rican independence, the end of forced sterilization of Puerto Rican women, health justice, and the improvement of the lives of Puerto Ricans as well as other racial minorities in mainland US through challenging institutionalized racism. Women formed more than half of the membership and were centrally involved in the organization, including Denise Oliver—who was a foremost figure of the group and appointed as the first woman in formal leadership in the group in 1970 (later also joining the Black Panther party), Iris Morales, Minerva Solla, Olguie Robles Toro, Gloria Rodriguez, and Connie Cruz. Since October 1969, gender equality was in the group's "Thirteen Point Program and Platform / Programa de 13 Puntos y Plataforma," which was written solely by the men of the group, indicating under the tenth point that "We Want Equality for Women. Machismo Must Be Revolutionary . . . Not Oppressive" (1970).[75] At the same time, while women were central to the group, they were not immune to sexism and had to fight for the party to incorporate feminism into its framework and question naturalized gender inequality. Specifically, the Young Lords Party was characterized by an uninterrogated chauvinism and machismo, with men in most leadership roles and women allotted more "feminized" positions such as secretarial work and child care. Male machismo was likewise tied to sexual assertiveness and compulsory sexuality, exhibited by the sexual objectification of women members—identified by women in the group as "sexual fascism."[76]

In response to prevailing sexism, 1970 saw the women of YLP—described affectionately by Oliver as "sister Lords"—undertake a Lysistrata-inspired politics of sexual refusal.[77] Forming a separate women's caucus and publishing a newspaper on gendered experiences in the organization, *La Luchadora,* the group complemented these organizational strategies with strategic political celibacy until all their demands were met by the central committee in June 1970.[78] The sex strike was effective in part because group members were forbidden from forming sexual relationships with nongroup members so as to prevent governmental infiltration. Writing on reproductive justice in the US, Jennifer Nelson relates that "the women's caucus [of the Young Lords Party] decided that it was time to force men in the Lords to take feminism seriously. . . . Influenced by Aristophenes' [sic] play, *Lysistrata,* they declared they would have no sexual relations with YLP men until the central committee met their demands, which included adding women to the central committee, elevating women to other positions of power, eradicating the call for revolutionary machismo from the platform, and integrating the defense committee by gender."[79] Other gains included increasing content on women and women's writing in *Palante,* making women's history central to the political education curriculum, developing child care for mothers who wanted to take part in YLP, forming a men's caucus to challenge sexism, and instigating the creation of a lesbian and gay caucus, of which famed transgender activist Sylvia Rivera was a member. Instituting a "no sex" strike in 1970 was a step that YLP's women members, including Oliver, took toward educating the group's members on sexism and implementing feminism into the structure of the organization. In turn, the YLP altered their Thirteen Point Program from "Machismo Must Be Revolutionary . . . Not Oppressive" (1970) to "Down with Machismo and Male Chauvinism" (1970) and held group members accountable for sexism.[80] In a position paper on women, they write, "We criticize those brothers who are 'machos' and who continue to treat our sisters as less than equals. . . . We are fighting every day within our PARTY against male chauvinism because we want to make a revolution of brothers and sisters—together—in love and respect for each other."[81] Drawing on this statement, the women in YLP drew on radical celibacy toward challenging systemic sexism so as to better fight racism. Building more equitability within the group, and formulating brothers and sisters as in pace with each other rather than in antagonistic deadlock, political celibacy constituted one tool that the Young Lords Party employed toward developing greater group cohesion and "wholeness" both for individual members and the group as a whole. Actively rooted in ending the desexualization of Puerto Rican women through coerced sterilization, the women of the Young Lords nonetheless envisioned a chosen, strategic, and temporary political celibacy as integral to effecting change within their organization.[82]

As Hill Collins has written, reflecting on Lorde's writing, "sexuality becomes a domain of restriction and repression when this energy is tied to the larger system of race, class, and gender oppression."[83] The antiracist celibacies I have discussed utilize a break from sex as a means of interrupting sexism and racism and of reasserting erotic wholeness and autonomy. In the National Young Lords Party's sex strike and Bambara's text, political celibacy/asexuality are voiced in terms that consider the specificities of what sexual refusal might mean for black women, women of color, and their political communities. Celibacy emerges as a suitable theoretical and organizing strategy for grappling with the intersections of gendered and racial injustice, creating more equitable relating between men and women, and building wholeness and autonomy both for individual men and women as for larger movements. Notably, and in differentiation to the celibacies I will next discuss, the goal, particularly with YLP's sex strike and Bambara's text, is not to create a separatist feminist space for women, but rather to use celibacy as a means to achieve greater cooperation and respect between men and women as a means to rally for the fight against white supremacy and racial injustice. While the gender binary is routinely invoked and assumptions are made about the categories of women and men, the overarching goal is working together rather than apart. Political celibacy/asexuality thus emerges as an antiracist tactic directed specifically at not only ending sexist oppression but as a step toward ending racist oppression as well.

## NIHILIST ASEXUALITY

Another stream of political celibacy/asexuality that emerged in the late sixties originates with the radical feminist uptake of Valerie Solanas's infamous *SCUM Manifesto* (1967).[84] Solanas was a radical antiestablishment figure, a sex worker, a sexual violence survivor, and poor—"theorizing and writing from the social gutter."[85] She intentionally disidentified from various identity positions, including feminism and lesbianism—rhetorically taking up nihilist asexuality as a radical challenge against the state, patriarchy, poverty, and basically everything she detested in the world. If erotics, as I formulated it at the outset of this chapter, is about the energy of collective struggle to end oppression, Solanas was on the outside of the erotic energies of the sixties and seventies since she worked as a single unit, alone against the system. Yet her work elucidates an acidic erotics that was based in a raging dissatisfaction with the conditions of her life. Applying a Lordean framework of erotics to Solanas, Solanas refused to be "docile and loyal and obedient, externally defined [and to] accept many facets of [her] oppression as [a] wom[a]n."[86] Instead, Solanas's erotics were based in a blistering anger against each and every condition of her own oppression and the erotic struggle to imagine a different futurity for those rare women she identified as "groovy." Further, Solanas's invective erotics provided a ground for the spurring of an asexual erotics among radical feminists, as I will explore in the subsequent sections.

While in recent years there has been a mounting interest in Solanas's antiestablishment persona, her work and her language have also been understood as transphobic. I read and understand Solanas as a radicalist who uses the *SCUM Manifesto* to disrupt hegemonic discourses of sexuality, writing from a position of a socially marginalized person who deploys against cisgender men many of the cultural myths that have been lodged against cisgender women throughout history. While, like many of the other feminists covered in this chapter, Solanas draws on a strong gender binary between "men"

and "women" and "males" and "females" as well as on biological determinism around gender, her work also at times undercuts this binary, suggesting
that in addition to men and women, she also envisions other genders such as
"groovy females," "scum women," and the "Men's Auxiliary" who defy patriarchy as well as "daddy's girls" and oppressive men who support patriarchy. In
this sense, it could be argued that she identifies several genders in her *SCUM
Manifesto*, even as she relies on the gender binary. Also, it should be noted that
Solanas herself did not give the name "The Society for Cutting Up Men" to her
manifesto—rather, it was provided by her publisher—and that the manifesto
itself was polemical rather than prescriptive.[87]

Borne of a frustration with the operations of prestige and wealth within a
patriarchal context that left her disinherited, impoverished, isolated, and living precariously on the inconsistent alms of others, Solanas's radical feminist
asexuality is a nihilistic asexuality, an asexuality of death, decay, and social
extermination—an antisocial thesis. Solanas speaks to us as a killjoy from
a position of nihilism, disbelieving in the possibility of change, even as she
advocates for a most radical type of system overthrow.[88] Her proposed solution
for overthrowing "male" society and culture is as follows. In the manifesto,
SCUM—who are "self-confident, swinging, thrill-seeking females"—are after
creating "a female society . . . [of] funky females grooving on each other."[89]
In order to do this, the true scum of the earth, or men who are oppressive,
must be eliminated in whatever way possible, and their "male culture" (i.e.,
patriarchy) must likewise be exterminated. Part of this strategy for eliminating
oppressive men is asexuality, an end to the reproduction of men. In addition
to aiding in the elimination of oppressive men, asexuality also redirects SCUM
women's attention to other pursuits, namely the remaking of society. SCUM
women are "those females least embedded in the male 'Culture,' the least nice,
those crass and simple souls who reduce fucking to fucking, who are . . . too
selfish to raise kids and husbands." Further, "these females are cool and rel-
atively cerebral and skirting asexuality."[90] Solanas writes that "if all women
simply left men, refused to have anything to do with them—ever, all men, the
government, and the national economy would collapse completely," and this
is the ambitious and fictitious goal of the *SCUM Manifesto*, a complete remaking of society through a complete annihilation of "male" (that is patriarchal,
capitalist) society and culture.[91] Crucially, asexuality is central to this, because
it fractures women's intimate ties with men, their oppressors, and thus frees
women to engage in the making of a new world and new world order. Women
do not have to bother with sex and they can adopt a post-sex politics since
"they've [already] seen the whole show—every bit of it—the fucking scene,
the sucking scene, the dyke scene—they've covered the whole waterfront,

been under every dock and pier—the peter pier, the pussy pier . . . you've got to go through a lot of sex to get to anti-sex, and SCUM's been through it all, and they're now ready for a new show; they want to crawl out from under the dock, move, take off, sink out."[92] In this sense, women can free up their energies, distance themselves from the efforts of pleasing others, seeking instead to "destroy the system, not attain certain rights within it."[93] This is a revolutionary vision that draws from Black Power organizing and efforts to build black culture apart from white people's control of culture and the ideology of white supremacy. For Solanas, this fictional project would involve the annihilation of any and all men who are oppressive, the end of the reproduction of male culture and gender, but also the end of reproduction itself, the end to the reproduction of the female gender and the cultural construction of femaleness. She asks, "Why produce even females? Why should there be future generations? What is their purpose?"[94] This nihilism serves to question the dominant patriarchal system as well as feminist stories of optimism, hope, and social repair. It is informed by Solanas's place on the margins of society and her inability to surmount the class-based and gender-based oppression in her own life as well as by a vision for a different world free of oppression.

It was Solanas's radical, and by that I mean unprecedented and ragingly angry text, along with the events that unfolded around her shooting of artist Andy Warhol, who functioned as a symbol of a "new" cultural capital that was nonetheless persistently male, white, and capitalist, that registered political celibacy/asexuality as a viable theoretical feminist tactic among radical feminists.[95] After Solanas's shooting of Warhol in 1968, Solanas became a contentious figure in feminist circles, with some touting her as a feminist symbol and others, such as the National Organization for Women (NOW), denouncing her violent actions as deleterious to the feminist movement and its public reception, with the NOW national president, Betty Friedan, arguing against the "sex warfare" of radical feminism.[96] Among Solanas's supporters, Flo Kennedy acted as her lawyer, Roxanne Dunbar-Ortiz visited her in jail, Ti-Grace Atkinson visited her in prison and attended her trial, and Robin Morgan (editor of Sisterhood Is Powerful [1970]), Dana Densmore, and Dunbar-Ortiz popularized her work in the women's movement.[97] Alice Echols, in Daring to Be Bad (1989), argues that Roxanne Dunbar-Ortiz introduced Solanas's text at the women's meeting that took place at Sandy Springs, Maryland, in August 1968, reading excerpts from the manifesto aloud and proclaiming it "the essence of feminism."[98] Shortly after, "SCUM . . . became obligatory reading for radical feminists," providing the basis for incorporating political celibacy/asexuality into radical feminist politics.[99]

## SEPARATIST CELIBACY

While Solanas's text was never univocally supported or upheld by radical feminists in the late 1960s, it did seem to serve as ground for inspiring further iterations of political celibacy/asexuality, especially among white feminists. Echols indicates that at the Lake Villa, Illinois conference, attended by over 200 women from thirty cities across the US and Canada, held Thanksgiving weekend in 1968 in line with the 120th anniversary of the first American women's right convention in Seneca Falls, celibacy emerged in a workshop on sex organized by two leading radical feminist figures: Anne Koedt (author of "The Myth of the Vaginal Orgasm" [1968]) with help from Ti-Grace Atkinson, former president of the New York NOW section.[100] During the workshop, Dana Densmore, a key radical feminist of the Boston radical feminist group Cell 16, advocated for women to practice celibacy rather than "squander their energy on men and sex."[101] Purportedly, there was disagreement and ambivalence over suggestions of political celibacy/asexuality, and some attendees, such as Amy Kesselman, were doubtful; Kesselman explained, "I didn't think that you could build a mass movement around celibacy. You have to promise people a better life, not a narrower life."[102]

Yet radical celibacy, in its separatist variety, nonetheless emerged as an implicit and explicit tactic in two radical feminist groups in particular—The Feminists and Cell 16. Unlike the political celibacy articulated by feminists of color and black feminists, which was intended to build stronger cohesion and wholeness between men and women toward antiracist struggle, separatist feminist groups employed political celibacy as a strategy of distancing from "movement men" in order to seek self-autonomy for mostly white women. This very different theorization and deployment of political celibacy/asexuality is directly grounded in a different experience of womanhood—notably, one where racism does not arise as a concern for white women—thereby facilitating the theorization of sexism as the basis from which all other injustice spurs. The erotics formulated here are grounded in self-autonomy, seeking self-knowledge and gender equality through a distancing from men and heterosexuality. Yet, even while articulating gender-based oppression as separate from race-based oppression, many radical feminist strategies were inspired by and drew on the tactics of the Black Power movement that members of these groups, and especially Ti-Grace Atkinson, were privy to through the bridge-building work of black feminists such as Flo Kennedy.[103]

The gender binary as well as biological determinism were central to feminist separatist politics even as the goal was to thwart ideas of what women were "supposed" to be, do, or look like. This involved seeing the world as divided between men, who were seen as acting in service of patriarchy and women's oppression, and women, who were oppressed by the patriarchal status quo through their reproductive facilities, the feminization of labor practices, domestic duties, lack of autonomy, beauty norms, and sex and heterosexuality. In this conceptualization, biology was sex and sex was gender in large part because that is how the feminists active in these groups experienced it. Further, heterosexuality and heterosexual sex were understood as colluding with the enemy. Separatism, in turn, modeled on Black Power organizing, was envisioned as an opportunity to start anew, apart from the muck of patriarchal oppression. This erotic project was rooted in the belief that women can form worlds and worldviews apart from patriarchy and gender oppression. In the words of Lorde, the erotic surfaces "as an assertion of the lifeforce of women; . . . [the] use of which we are now reclaiming in our language, our history, our dancing, our loving, our work, our lives."[104] Under feminist separatism, each part of life was utilized toward seeking an antisexist erotic—from shelter making and building communities to activist work and political organizing. These erotics were grounded in a critical approach to sexism and heterosexuality as well as in the thrill of organizing with other women, or in Lorde's words, "the power which comes from sharing deeply any pursuit with another person" and in "examin[ing] the ways in which [the] world can be truly different."[105] Separatism had at its heart a desire to imagine and build a nonpatriarchal world through the formation of erotic affinities between women, with political celibacy/asexuality facilitating this building.

The Feminists, originally called the October 17th Movement, were a New York–based group formed when Ti-Grace Atkinson and Flo Kennedy split from NOW in 1968.[106] As Randolph discusses, due in large part to the work of Kennedy, who was involved in antiracist struggles, the roots of the split from NOW and the formation of the new group were linked—at least at first—to a more intersectional agenda that saw the women's movement in relation to the student movement and the black freedom movement.[107] The October 17th Movement also included black writer and producer Kay Lindsey (who published a poem in Bambara's *The Black Woman*), and white feminists Charlotte Hill, Nanette Rainone, Carol Goodman, and Astrid Bergundaugen.[108] In 1969 the organization changed its name to The Feminists, which it used until its breakup in 1973, and developed a focus on male supremacy as the root of all other forms of oppression. While Kennedy appreciated the group's separatism, she, Lindsey, and other black feminists left the group because it focused too narrowly on sexism apart from racism.[109]

The Feminists developed a critique of the institution of heterosexuality that included an implicit tendency, at least theoretically, toward political celibacy/asexuality. Focusing on gender as the primary form of oppression and overlooking the intersections of gender and race, The Feminists advocated that heterosexuality functions to bind women to reproduction and mothering, such as through the myth of the vaginal orgasm or the willful ignorance of the clitoral orgasm.[110] They espoused an early vanguard separatism, which either transferred sexual pleasure to autoeroticism and masturbation or implicitly called for celibacy from men. The Feminists even developed rules around how many women in the group could remain married to men (one third), understanding marriage as collaboration with the enemy, and "rejecting marriage and fidelity to the male."[111]

Sexual intercourse was framed by the group as a "social act" that provides men with the opportunity to assert power over women and thus to maintain women in subservience to men; political celibacy/asexuality—that is, a denial of sex to men—was a way to establish self-autonomy and work toward the abolishment of the sex-caste system.[112] For instance, in "The Institution of Sexual Intercourse" (1970), Atkinson writes, "society has never known a time when sex in all its aspects was not exploitative and relations based on sex, e.g., the male-female relationship, were not extremely hostile, it is [thus] difficult to understand how sexual intercourse can . . . be salvaged as a practice."[113] However, lesbian sex was also repudiated since "lesbians, by definition, accept that human beings are primarily sexual" and thus "in some sense, inferior."[114] Echols draws on an interview with Irene Peslikis (briefly a member of The Feminists), who indicated that the point "wasn't to give up men for women, it was just to give it up!"[115] In this way, informed by Solanas's nihilist asexuality and by the strategies of Black Power, political celibacy/asexuality emerged for The Feminists as an implicit strategy for women to separate from male demands on their bodies and to redefine themselves as something other than *the sex*.[116] The energy, love, and time that would have been funneled into caring for one's man was instead directed at other women in the group, since "feminists must strive to love each other and not be confused with the distractions that sex offers."[117] Sex, if any, was to be had with men through an approach of "amazon virginity," that is, an emotionally uninvested sex that did not take itself seriously.[118]

Another radical feminist group that explicitly advocated for political celibacy/asexuality was the Boston group Cell 16, formed in 1968 by Roxanne Dunbar-Ortiz, and which included Dana Densmore, Jeanne Lafferty, Lisa Leghorn, Abby Rockefeller, Betsy Warrior, and Jayne West. While most of the group members were white, Dunbar-Ortiz has since identified as Indigenous and works as an Indigenous historian. As is evident in the journal they produced, *No More Fun and Games: A Journal of Female Liberation* (1968–1973), Cell 16 partook in separatism and an explicit and radical sexual abstinence.[119] Cell 16, similar to The Feminists, developed a vanguard separatist politics that involved all-female communal living; a particular aesthetic style consisting of short hair, khakis, combat boots, and work shirts; a commitment to self-sufficiency; training in karate as a means of cultivating bodily autonomy and self protection; and a theoretical and practical political celibacy/asexuality.[120] Political separatist celibacy emerged as a sustained theme in pursuit of "destroy[ing] the three pillars of class (caste) society—the family, private property, and the state—and their attendant evils—corporate capitalism, imperialism, war, racism, misogyny, annihilation of the balance of nature."[121] While racism is formulated here alongside misogyny, the groundwork for social transformation is rooted in theorizing gender-based oppression and the ways it is upheld through men's sexual access to women.

Separatist celibacy was here a practice and theory of disengaging, emotionally and politically, from men and male systems of oppression and a creative project of imagining worlds without men. While aspects of the politics, ethos, and practice of the group shifted over time, a separatist celibacy/asexuality remained integral to Cell 16's staking of bodily autonomy and collective identity. In many ways, the political celibacy/asexuality that emerged is resonant with what is understood today as "aromanticism," though it was a politically motivated aromanticism that sought to assert women as rational agents not dependent on men for emotional support or touch-based bonding. In Densmore's words, "Happy, healthy, self-confident animals and people don't like being touched, don't need to snuggle and huggle. . . . They are really free and self-contained and in their heads."[122]

Throughout *No More Fun and Games* (*NMFG*), but especially in several keys pieces—including Densmore's "On Celibacy" (*NMFG* 1, 1968/1970) and "Independence from the Sexual Revolution" (1971); Dunbar-Ortiz's "Asexuality" (*NMFG* 1, 1968/1970) and "'Sexual Liberation': More of the Same Thing" (*NMFG* 3, 1969); Ellen O'Donnell's "Thoughts on Celibacy" (*NMFG* 1, 1968/1970); and Indra Allen's "Why I Am Celibate" (*NMFG* 6, 1973)—compulsory sexuality is undermined, challenging the notion that sex is a natural, bodily need that has been rendered central to the self by a patriarchal culture invested in keeping women's bodies sexually available for men.[123] For instance, in "On Celibacy" (1968/1970), Densmore combats the slipping of sex into health and health into sex, writing that "sex is not essential to life, as eating is. Some people go through their whole lives without engaging in it at all, including fine, warm, happy people. It is a myth that this makes one bitter, shriveled up, twisted."[124] In this way, Densmore challenged the figuration of sex as acontextually "healthy" or "good" as well as the pathologization of so-called frigidity. Also, in "Independence from the Sexual Revolution" (1971), she questions the efficacy of equating sex with freedom, sardonically asserting that "sex becomes a religion" and that "it's forced down our throats."[125] She writes that "people seem to believe that sexual freedom . . . is freedom" and complains it is a "sexual freedom that includes no freedom to decline sex."[126] Through such commentary, Densmore desutures sex from ideas of "freedom" and "liberation" and predates Foucault's analysis of the discourse of sex as "liberatory." In her suspicion of 1960s free-love conflations of sex and freedom, she draws attention to the disciplinary and regulatory forces of sexuality. Further, Densmore questions whether sex is really that much more exciting and pleasurable than other activities, decentering the specialness of sex, writing that "a lot of things are pleasurable without our getting the idea that we can't live without them. . . . I can think of certain foods, certain music, certain drugs, whose physical pleasurableness compares favorably even to good sex."[127] Also, Densmore questions the coital and penis-centered teleological narrative of heterosexual sex. She writes, "we *feel* that we need sex, but the issue is very confused. What is it we really need? Is it orgasms? Intercourse? Intimacy with another human being? Stroking? Companionship? Human kindness? And do we 'need' it physically or psychologically?"[128] Using the strategy of raising questions, Densmore alludes to the many binds that hold sex in high esteem socioculturally: a particular androcentric narrative invested in heterosexual sex, an orgasmic and coital imperative, the "fallacy of misplaced scale," the conflation of sex and health, the sexual imperative and compulsory sexuality, and the very unclear quality of what "sex" and "sexuality" actually include and on whose terms.[129] In this way, Densmore raises many of the points that have since been theorized by queer theory, critical sexuality studies, and asexuality studies, providing one of the first critical interjections into liberatory sex discourse.[130]

Amidst this critique of sex's disciplinary functions, celibacy/asexuality emerges as both an analytic for studying sex in patriarchal contexts and as a practice that can disrupt women's emotional, sexual, and social dependence on men, encouraging autonomy, independence, and bonds with other women instead. In "On Celibacy" Densmore rallies: "This is a call not for celibacy but for an acceptance of celibacy as an honorable alternative, one preferable to the degradation of most male-female sexual relationships. But it is only when we accept the idea of celibacy completely that we will ever be able to liberate ourselves."[131] Densmore advances that sex is time-absorbing for women because of all the grooming, flirting, and preparations that lead up to it, diverting time away from women's liberation.[132] Thus "many girls who would be most free to fight in the female liberation struggle are squandering valuable energy."[133] In this context, celibacy is celebrated as an optimistic, efficacious strategy for women to gain independence from men and funnel time and energy toward women instead. As a hopeful feminist asexual story, Cell 16's celibate feminism lubricates readers for the feminist revolution, encouraging women to use their bodies and time as tools against the hetero-patriarchal regime. In this sense, gender oppression is envisioned as a struggle undertaken by women separate from men, without accounting for the ways in which women of color battle simultaneously with sexism and racism.

Cell 16's as well as The Feminists' separatist celibacy was bound to a gender-based separatism, with the goal of forming erotic communities devoid of sex, thus freeing up energy for other political pursuits and for the assertion of a self-sufficient self. Sisterhood here took the form of a distinctly asexual variety, in pursuit of building erotic and political bonds outside of sex and the sexual apparatus. Well-known lesbian novelist and feminist Rita Mae Brown indicates, in *A Plain Brown Rapper* (1976), that when she challenged Cell 16 for their inattentiveness to lesbianism, Dunbar-Ortiz responded: "What I want to do is to get women out of bed. Women can love each other but they don't have to sleep together."[134] In my reading, while inattentive to lesbian sex, Cell 16 and The Feminists were nonetheless involved in forming erotically lesbian feminist asexual communities since they avidly committed themselves to channeling energy toward other women. What makes Cell 16's and The Feminists' lesbian feminism distinct is their additional commitment to celibacy/asexuality both among their members and in regard to men. In other words, Cell 16 and The Feminists practiced and theorized a political celibacy/asexuality as a radical boycott against patriarchal relations and systems that saw women, first and foremost, as existing for men, while also engaging in an asexual, aromantic sisterly erotics between themselves. That this lesbian feminist utopian project did not involve sex does not make it nonlesbian or unerotic. "Sisterhood felt good" for these women, but it was an asexual sisterhood that imagined celibacy/asexuality as an effective strategy for both removing their labors from men and for building a community with each other. Separatist celibacy/asexuality constituted a form of erotic engagement that would become central to feminist organizing in the late sixties and early seventies in that it formed the groundwork for employing asexuality as a method to foster erotics between women, forming the basis for lesbian feminist communities.

## LESBIAN CELIBACY

The final political celibacy/asexuality I will consider is that of lesbian celibacy, which was central to early lesbian feminist articulations of separatism. Rita

Mae Brown, who also penned the well-read lesbian novel *Rubyfruit Jungle* (1973), along with Charlotte Bunch and others, organized in 1971 one of the leading lesbian feminist collectives of the era, The Furies, which focused on communal living, feminist politics, and separatism.[135] Lesbian feminism took off after the Lavender Menace action organized by the New York–based group, Radicalesbians, at the Second Congress to Unite Women on May 1, 1970, at which "The Woman Identified Woman" paper—which identified lesbianism as based on bonds between women rather than on sex between women—was distributed.[136] Addressing the homophobia in the women's movement, the action consisted of women in "lavender menace"–stenciled T-shirts taking control of the stage and engaging in a two-hour discussion that sought to legitimize lesbianism through arguing that it was not solely a "bedroom issue."[137] Lesbianism emerged in this historical moment less as a sexual orientation and more as a political choice, a political strategy integral to feminist organizing and to the separatist energy of forming communities outside of male supremacy. As Ginny Berson of The Furies wrote, "Lesbianism is not a matter of sexual preference, but rather one of political choice which every woman must make if she is to become woman-identified and thereby end male supremacy."[138] Lesbianism became central to feminism and it became, as Echols identifies it, the "quintessential act of political solidarity with other women."[139] With the goal of imagining a feminist politics that seeped into all elements of life practice and challenged male supremacy, an erotic and asexually infused lesbian feminism was born.

The Furies, based in Washington, DC, drew on the energies of The Feminists' and Cell 16's distancing from sex, explorations of alternative life practices, and queer questioning of heterosexual coupling. Comprised solely of white women of working-class and middle-class backgrounds, The Furies focused on sex-based oppression as it related to class-based oppression and the oppression of lesbians. They published a lesbian newspaper, *The Furies* (1972–1973), and developed communal lesbian living strategies based on a socialist pooling of resources.[140] In practice and theory, The Furies saw sexism as the root of all oppression, wanting to see the end of lesbians' and women's oppression as a strategy for also undoing capitalism, imperialism, and racism.[141]

Crucially, lesbianism was identified as a political orientation and not as something that was fundamentally about sex or sexual desire for women. The newspaper itself never included poetry or fiction about sex or images of nudity so as to challenge the idea that lesbianism is only about sex.[142] The desire, instead, was for an erotic coming together with other women toward challenging sexist and homophobic society—it was the desire for revolution.

Channeling energy away from men and toward other women and feminist organizing fed fluidly into a lesbianism laced with asexuality, wherein feminists formed erotic bonds with each other that did not always include sex and did not focus on sexual desire.

Lesbian feminism was thus potent with political celibacy/asexuality. Because sex was deemphasized both to gain credibility for lesbianism within the feminist movement and also because sex was understood in part as in service of the hetero-patriarchal regime, lesbianism was not bound to a sexual practice or sexual desire; it was a tool for freeing women from sexism. If anything, lesbian feminism was articulated in distinction to sex and as sensuality. For example, Sue Katz wrote:

> For me, coming out meant an end to sex. It's dead and gone in my life. I reject that institution totally. Sex means oppression, it means exploitation. . . . Physical contact and feelings have taken a new liberatory form, and we call that "sensuality" . . . gay feminism now is a fantastically sensual experience for me. . . . Physicalness is now a creative non-institutionalized experience. It is touching and rubbing and cuddling and fondness. . . . Its only goal is closeness and pleasure. It does not exist for the Big Orgasm. It exists for feeling nice. Our sensuality may or may not include genital experience . . . There is no set physical goal to our sensuality. There is no sex. The whole language is oppressive. It is white male-oriented and heterosexual. . . . Sensuality is formless and amorphous. It can grow and expand as we feel it. . . . The sensuality I feel has transformed my politics, has solved the contradiction between my mind and my body because the energies for our feminist revolution are the same as the energies of our love for women.[143]

Katz indicates here, first, the rejection of sex as an institution that she associated with keeping hetero-patriarchy alive. While it could be argued that Katz is simply arguing for lesbian sex as opposed to sex in straight contexts, she is also gesturing to something bigger, broader—an erotics. She grounds erotics in sensuality, in creative and not necessarily sex-based forms for relating to others intimately. These erotics are about the feeling of revolution grounded in spending time with other women toward building communities of resistance. Erotics surface here as rooted in a praxis of asexuality/celibacy that enabled vital erotic energy for other pursuits, including the making of a revolution. Or, as Sue Negrin describes: "gay feminism [was] the only space in which to develop nonsexual sensuality."[144] As such, lesbianism was being argued on asexual grounds, not necessarily desexualized so much as imagined beyond sex, which was associated with coercive, exploitative, and nonpleasurable hetero-patriarchy. Speaking broadly to a dissatisfaction with sex—its meaning, practice, and social function—the origins of lesbian feminism and women's communes of the era were imagined, in part, as a break from sex:

> We have been taught that sexual relationships are the primary form of human relations. . . . Many women have become alienated from the sexual functions of their bodies because sex has been used to keep us in our place. As a step toward wholeness, mustn't we withdraw from the oppression of sexual mindfucks and build all female collectives? Some may include sex between women, but for many, these collectives will probably be a period of celibacy—probably the first time in most women's lives.[145]

Invoking "wholeness" in a way parallel to the antiracist celibacies I examined earlier, celibacy is articulated as a means for gaining self-knowledge and, drawing on Lorde, increased awareness of one's erotic powers. Celibacy emerges as a distinct practice for erotic self-knowledge, for breaking with hetero-patriarchy, as well as an opportunity for redirecting one's erotic energies to relationships with women. An ulterior sensuality emerges in these accounts that is informed by political celibacy/asexuality and resonant with an erotics intent on exploring other forms of intimacy between bodies than sex per se, and other bonding energies than sexual desire. The desires of these articulations of sisterhood are in excess of sex and sexual desire and are permeated with a politically motivated asexual erotics. While critiques of lesbian feminism commonly assert that lesbianism was desexualized or sanitized so as to make it more palatable, or that it was in fact all about lesbian sex at its core, I am suggesting that this does not account for the feeling flows that informed lesbian feminist formation. Asexuality and celibacy facilitated erotics and lesbianism rather than preventing either. While there was certainly a strategic advantage to be gained from making lesbianism less about sex and more about feminism in that it made lesbianism more palatable politically in a homophobic historical context, the crucial insight is that sex and feminism were somehow felt as distinct from one another, and that asexual lesbianism traveled further, affectively speaking, among feminist women, than a strictly sexual and sex-based lesbianism could have. In this sense, lesbian feminism is informed not only by the political celibacy/asexuality of groups such as The Feminists and Cell 16 but also by the very feeling that somehow, inexplicably, something about sisterhood felt asexual. Erotics emerge here as not bound to and by sexual desire but as grounded in the energy of women being together away and apart from heterosexuality. Women were drawn to each other erotically rather than strictly sexually in the pursuit of carving out revolutionary worlds. Political celibacy and political asexuality, in turn, facilitated the development of a lesbian erotics.

## SISTERHOOD FEELS ASEXUAL

Lorde wrote that "the celebration of the erotic" is "a longed for bed which [one] enter[s] gratefully and from which [one] rise[s] up empowered."[146] In this sense, the bed featured on the poster with which I opened this chapter is suggestive of the power of erotics contained within political celibacy and political asexuality in the sixties and seventies. As a strategy mobilized by feminists of color toward the greater good of antiracist struggles, by Solanas and radical feminists toward unmaking sexism, and by lesbian feminists toward fuelling the erotics of relating between women, political asexuality/celibacy emerged as a set of complex and vital practices of resistance. That today is a time when asexuality, as a sexual identity, is slowly gaining in credibility and acceptance, as is demonstrated by the rise in asexuality research and activisms, further speaks to the necessity of examining what is at stake in ignoring political celibacies/asexualities. Political asexuality/celibacy, while often understood as a form of "anti-sex," constituted an energizing practice and theory that fostered, rather than impeded, erotic development in the sixties and seventies, fueling the erotics of revolutionary action for feminists. As an integral part of the energy of movement organizing in an era radiant with feminist and antiracist momentum, political celibacies/asexualities were a key theory and technique for deepening and strengthening the erotic power of revolution.

# CHAPTER 2

# Lesbian Bed Death, Asexually

## *An Erotics of Failure*

MAKING ITS ROUNDS through social networks' lesbian channels, an article from *Archer Magazine,* an Australian magazine of sexual diversity, blazes the headline "The Era of Lesbian Bed Death Is Over, Long Live Lesbian Fuck Eye." The piece reads, "today . . . lesbian women have more orgasms, better sex and sex that lasts longer than their heterosexual female counterparts. And they've also mastered Lesbian Fuck Eye."[1] Striving to celebrate lesbianism, the piece seeks to creatively replace one memorable trope of lesbianism, lesbian bed death, with another—"an eye that embodies sexual desire and identity in one fell swoop."[2] It marks what it designates as a pivotal moment in lesbian culture, a move away from the moribund desexualizing tendencies of lesbian bed death, with its baggage of failure and sexual attrition, and toward the hopeful horizon of sex and sexual desire. In this chapter, I seek to analyze the attachment of lesbianism to sexual desire through a reverse reading focused on the erotics of lesbian bed death. Whereas in the previous chapter I looked at how political asexuality/celibacy were central tenets of feminist erotics in the 1960s and 1970s, in this chapter I consider how fears of asexuality inform lesbian erotics.

Lesbian bed death arose as an idiomatic shorthand at the hands of the therapeutic model of sexual functioning. Routinely attributed, as an observable phenomenon, to sociologists Pepper Schwartz and Philip Blumstein from their 1983 book *American Couples,* it is a term imbued with layers of gendered, lesbian-skeptical, and sexunormative ideals of sexual functioning.[3] Less overtly, it is also attached to ideals of white, middle-class, able-bodied productivity. It houses dreams and hopes of the good life and the fears and anxieties that are attached to its loss. I unpack the operations of lesbian bed death, assessing that what is ultimately at stake in this pernicious idiom is an overburdening of sex with salutary, promissory qualities unrivalled by other activities and forms of relating. The promises of sex are manifold and specific to various contexts. Sex promises love and pleasure, and it also promises a particular way of life, a narrative of health and success in a neoliberal regime of desire bound up with ideals of the good life, the white middle-class life, the coupled and reproductive life. Overrun by such promises, sex thus also becomes a site of anxiety, an anxiety that if one fails at its performance, one will lose the trappings of the good life. As Lauren Berlant and Lee Edelman argue, "sex gets invested with such a weighty burden of optimism *as well as* with an often overwhelming burden of anxiety."[4] Lesbian bed death's continued presence in lesbian representation, as I will explore, indexes an anxiety around the loss of the promise of sex, which has only recently been extended to lesbians through the public recognition and acceptance of lesbian coupled formations.

Thinking through the anxieties attached to lesbian bed death, I reimagine lesbian bed death as an erotics of failure, an asexual erotics that homes in on social investments in sex. Failing both asexuality and lesbianism, in the sense that it makes an absence of sex into a pathologized, morose, and moribund condition, lesbian bed death nonetheless provides a versatile trope for studying lesbian fears of asexuality. It offers the ground for a particular type of erotics that I will explore as "asexuality without optimism."[5]

Because "there is a myth that *still* clings to lesbian sex: that of the dreaded Lesbian Bed Death, or, the idea that lesbians shack up and then stop having sex," and because there is a parallel myth that clings to a lack of sex as a dreaded state, I find it necessary to offer an asexual reading of lesbian bed death.[6] In this way, the goal of this chapter is to read lesbian bed death from an asexual perspective that does not try to repatriate sex into lesbianism, but rather asks why such a project is at all necessary. Tracking the concept of lesbian bed death, or LBD, I begin this chapter through a contextualizing of both the advent of lesbian bed death and its feminist and queer critiques, providing a review of the literature on lesbian bed death. The subsequent three sections play with the three-word moniker lesbian-bed-death by offering up asexually invested explorations of each of these three terms and their function as a unit. In "Lesbian," I turn to mainstream television and film representations of lesbianism to demonstrate that while commonly rejected, lesbian bed death tends to inform the parameters of the popular imagining of lesbian representation. In particular, a whole host of mainstreamed shows and films, including *Orange Is the New Black, The Fosters, The Kids Are All Right,* and *The L Word,* demonstrate their anxiety around lesbian bed death and what it metonymizes for lesbian identity in general. Yet, while asexuality is invoked only by way of anxiety around LBD in these representations, it nonetheless has a vivid history within lesbian writing, including through work focused on Boston marriages, intimate friendships, the woman-identified-woman of lesbian feminism, and lesbian and queer trauma. In "Bed," I turn to the genre of lesbian art, created by and for lesbian-identified people, providing an asexual analysis of two bed-centered photographic series, Tammy Rae Carland's *Lesbian Beds* (2002) and *Lesbian Bedrooms II* (2011) by Kyle Lasky. I do so by situating both series in the context of artistic engagements with the bed as a form of politicized commentary, studying the asexual aesthetic undercurrents of each series. Finally, in "Death," I draw on queer affect studies to argue for the affective utility of an erotics of failure, an asexual analysis that is not attached to celebratory identity rhetoric but that rather refuses optimism.

## LESBIAN BED DEATH: A SHORT HISTORY

Lesbian bed death arises as a phenomenon out of Pepper Schwartz and Philip Blumstein's 1983 book *American Couples: Money, Work, Sex,* feeding off their empirical evidence to suggest that women in long-term lesbian relationships have lower rates of sexual activity than other coupled populations, such as married straight couples, cohabiting straight couples, and gay male couples.[7] Schwartz and Blumstein write that their "research shows that lesbians have a lower sexual frequency at every stage of a relationship, at every point in their lives."[8] The causal factors provided for lower frequency of sex are situated in terms of socialization. The authors argue that because men are socialized to be sexually aggressive and women to be sexually passive, a relationship with two women leads to a surplus of sexual passivity, thus forming the ground for a hesitancy toward sexual initiation.[9] Another motivation provided for lower rates of sex is the idea of "fusion" or "merging," or that because women are socialized to be relational, within a relationship they easily fuse into one unit, making the expressiveness of sexual intimacy unnecessary.[10] Concern over lesbian bed death gained momentum within lesbian-affirmative sex therapy of the 1990s and became a key site of investigation within the therapeutic literature.[11] Ultimately Schwartz and Blumstein's study, and others that followed on its heels or developed along similar lines, not only put forward what has been commonly understood as a damaging idea of lesbians as desexualized and of women as sexually passive, but also sedimented the notion that a good sex life, measured by frequency of sexual encounters, is integral to a loving, healthy relationship.

Yet Schwartz and Blumstein's and similar work has been effectively critiqued by lesbian and feminist scholars for "a privileging of male definitions of sexuality, and a perpetuation of myths and attitudes about female sexuality."[12] Kristina Gupta argues that from its advent, the concept was criticized as well as disproved.[13] More recently, Jacqueline Cohen and Sandra Byers, in a 2014 study of 586 women in same-sex relationships of one to thirty-six years in length, found that regardless of relationship duration, most women continued to partake in genital and nongenital sexual behaviors about once a week.[14]

Clinical sexologist Michele O'Mara, frustrated with the lack of transparency as to the phrase's origin and the common misattribution of the phrase itself to Schwartz and Blumstein, argued that the phrase "lesbian bed death" formed spontaneously among lesbians in the mid- to later 1980s because it spoke to a common experience.[15] O'Mara demonstrates not only that it has a collective lesbian history of emergence as a satirical term but also that it embeds within it a lesbian sex-positive critique of sexual absence, since Jade McGleughlin, credited with its first open usage, "wanted the sexiness of talking about sex" and "LBD included more than the diminishing sex in a lesbian's personal relationship . . . [as] it also captured the larger loss of a sexual community."[16] In other words, lesbians invented the phrase "lesbian bed death" as a loving term to critically think about the social derision of lesbianism.

Critiques of lesbian bed death, such as psychologist and sex therapist Suzanne Iasenza's, outline that the reliance on Schwartz and Blumstein's study as evidence for lesbian bed death is unreliable since their data is flawed. First, while many studies provided evidence contrary to theirs, Schwartz and Blumstein became cited so often that a large body of literature has been built on their findings alone.[17] Also, Iasenza argues that upon a careful reading of Schwartz and Blumstein, it is not altogether clear whether they found that lesbians are, in fact, less sexually active than other coupled formations but only that the type of sex they are having might not qualify under popular schemas of hetero-coital sex, since their study used "male-defined measurements of sex that misrepresent the subjective experiences of women" through placing a premium on frequency and genital sex as opposed to on quality.[18] Cohen and Byers's more recent study, which collected evidence that disproves the existence of LBD, for instance, challenges restrictive models of both sex and sexual identification by including nongenital sexual activities, sexual satisfaction measures, and individuals who are in same-sex relationships but who do not identify as "lesbians."[19] Schwartz and Blumstein, in distilling lesbian relationships to patterns of socialization—that is, in saying that lesbians are socialized to be sexually passive—"may have simply traded a biopsychological essentialism in for a biosocial essentialism" without regard for how other social vectors, such as ability, age, class, race, butchness/femmemness, and asexuality shape lesbian practices and relations.[20]

Lesbian bed death is thus a trope with specific attachments to heteronormative discourses of gender, sexuality, and sexunormativity. While its phraseology is in part sarcastic and embeds a sex-positive critique of sexual decline, clinically, lesbian bed death has been used as a trope to sediment lesbians into a homogenous population overscripted by their gendered socialization in terms of passivity.[21] As a trope, lesbian bed death comes to honor particular commitments to gender that rest on a gender binary system and biological determinism, within which women and men are understood both as discrete and distinct entities and as homogenously characterized by particular features. While men are conceived of as sexual aggressors who are interested in sex on straightforward and teleological terms, women are positioned as sexually passive and unwilling to initiate sex as a consequence of their socialization. In this sense, lesbian bed death comes to the fore to sediment particular gendered relations, so that even while it purports to be descriptive of the group "lesbians," it smuggles in a two-gendered system of proper sexual conduct— entrenching passivity among women and sexual activeness among men and reinscribing the possibility of only two genders and paths of socialization.

Further, as Iasenza, Gupta, and others have demonstrated, lesbian bed death, as it is elaborated by clinical literature, functions to desexualize lesbians and lesbian relating in a context where the enactment of sex speaks to the worth, value, and vitality of a person and relationship.[22] Desexualization is here a phenomenon distinct from asexuality in that it imposes an absence of sex and sexuality not as an erotic possibility but as a biopolitical strategy, dispensing the promise of sex only to those who are understood as having a right to it. Sex is a promise unevenly distributed, and its salutary qualities are most frequently granted to white, middle-class, able-bodied, and heterosexual populations, which are understood as socially valuable.

In this sense, the trope of lesbian bed death speaks exactingly to sexunormativity, or the complex system of habits and discourses that encourages us to perform on sexual terms.[23] As a pejorative phrase, "lesbian bed death" attaches itself to fears around the loss of sex and sexuality and what this comes to signify for belonging, relational formations, self-actualization, and futurity. As a term, it functions in a disciplinary sense to discourage both lesbianism (purported as the site of sex's death) and to enforce sexual repatriation at any cost.

Thus, many of the critiques of lesbian bed death, including the "Lesbian Fuck Eye" provocation in *Archer Magazine,* are aimed toward demonstrating that lesbians do in fact have great sex, that this sex is as good as if not better than straight sex, and that lesbian bed death is a "myth," a "fallacy."[24] In other words, these critiques continue to flesh out an attachment to sex as the life force of a romantic relationship, and they are infused with anxieties around a loss of sex. This leads to a neglect of the asexual erotics within lesbian identification, representation, and theory. Even within Schwartz and Blumstein's rendition of lesbian sexual failure, there are nodes of asexuality that have been set aside in the push to disprove lesbian bed death. For instance, they cite one participant who clearly articulates her need for nonsexual intimacies in a way that is resonant with asexuality. The participant indicates: "I started feeling like all she wanted to do was be in bed, and I started feeling like that was taking away from everything else in our relationship. It snowballed into me feeling, like, well, I don't even want that anymore if we can't talk and we can't do anything else together."[25] As I will elaborate later in this chapter, such instances of asexuality become occluded in the hunt to prove that lesbianism is sexual.

Crucially, lesbian bed death provides an asexual current of lesbian sexuality, directing us to instances when asexuality might be present but is misnamed and pathologized. On the one hand, LBD is commonly critiqued and demolished as a myth rooted in sexist and homophobic assumptions about lesbian relationships. On the other hand, lesbian bed death lives on in the cultural imaginary and is regularly resuscitated in representations of lesbians. That lesbian bed death refuses to die suggests not that it is a true occurrence but rather that it is a true anxiety. Lesbian bed death, as a phenomenon to be contested, is also imbued with its own ideals as to which lesbians are being desexualized and which lesbians should be repatriated into sexual life. Namely, lesbian bed death is a cultural trope that is fought against most vociferously in middle-class, white, able-bodied, and neoliberal contexts, as the examples I will next consider flesh out.

## LESBIAN: LESBIAN BED DEATH ON SCREEN

To better render lesbian bed death as an appellation of anxiety around the loss of sex, I turn to several mainstream cultural representations, tracking the promise of sex and the failure of lesbian bed death. In particular, while there has been a host of representations of lesbian bed death, including in Alison Bechdel's *Dykes to Watch Out For* as well as in the TV shows *Orange Is the New Black, The Fosters,* and *The L Word* and the film *The Kids Are All Right,* I will focus on two representations of lesbian bed death, in the ABC television series *The Fosters* and in Lisa Cholodenko's film *The Kids Are All Right*.[26] I have decided to focus on these two representations because they effectively help us understand how ideals of lesbian sex are affiliated with a particular form of white, middle-class-aspiring, able-bodied homo-citizenship. They are also both examples of a "mainstreamed lesbianism" that has come to function as in itself a sign of progress, speaking to the making palatable of queer desire under a homonormative agenda.[27] Far from the politically motivated lesbian feminism we saw in the last chapter, this lesbianism is socially desirable and as naturally all-American as the white picket-fenced family.

*The Fosters* is an American TV drama first launched in 2013 on the ABC Family Network and stretching across five seasons. It centers around the life of a not exactly heteronormative but stubbornly upper-middle-class and neoliberal family consisting of an interracial lesbian couple, police officer Stef (played by Teri Polo) and vice principal at a secondary school Lena (played by Sherri Saum), and their family of adopted, fostered, and biological children—Jesus and Mariana, Callie and Jude, and Brandon. Together the Fosters form an unusual family unit that breaks in several ways from normative notions of the reproductive family. They are headed by two lesbian parents, multiracial (Stef, Brandon, Callie, and Jude are presumably white, Lena is black, Jesus and Mariana are Latinx), from disaggregate class backgrounds, and fluid in formation (since initially Callie and Jude are not legally adopted but rather are being "fostered" in both senses of the term). At the same time, the family is framed as an upstanding one by American standards. Securely middle class, with careers in law and justice and education, Stef and Lena are portrayed as a solid, unshakeable formation, firm but kind, loving, and incredibly secure in their sense of themselves, their place in the world, and their ability to share their good life with children in the foster care system.

Crucially, their good life, their obvious membership in the community of productive workers and a loving family is entangled in their ability to stave off lesbian bed death and through doing so to maintain the integrity of their loving couplehood. Michael Cobb, in his book *Single: Arguments for the Uncoupled* (2012), explores how the couple formation rests on ideals of monogamy and surfaces as a dominant relational model in contemporary contexts, pushing other forms of relating—including friendship networks, polyamory, and especially the single life—into the gutter.[28] The couple, married or unmarried, straight or gay, continues to form the pillar of capitalist models of self-actualization under the rubrics of the good life. To be single in this schema is to have the care, energy, and love of others withdrawn from you, to be rendered secondary to the integrity of the couple.[29] Sex plays a central, though certainly

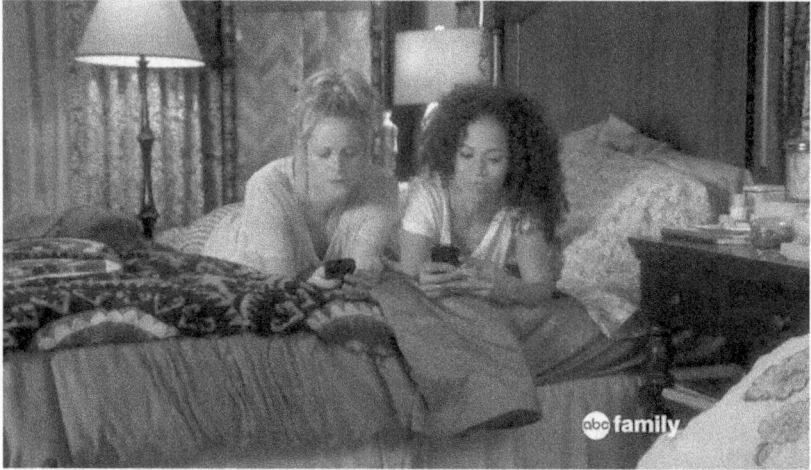

**FIGURE 2.1.** Still from season 1 of *The Fosters*. Stef (left) and Lena (right) plan a sex date on their smartphones.

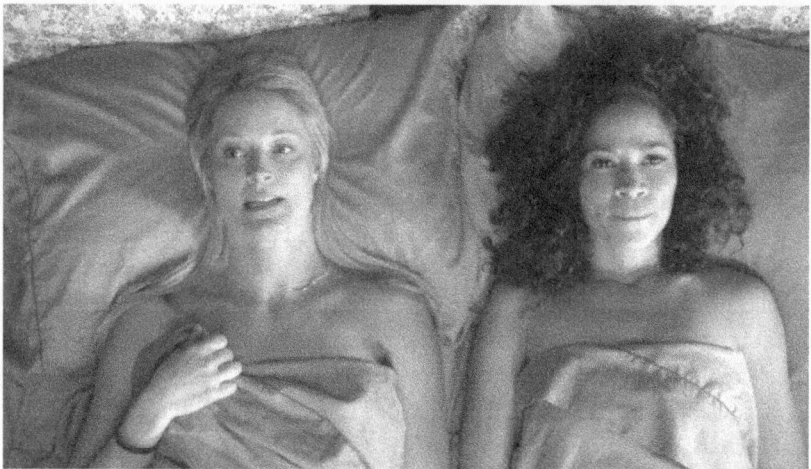

**FIGURE 2.2.** Still from season 2 of *The Fosters*. Stef (left) and Lena (right) undergoing "lesbian bed death."

not exclusive role here in the sedimenting of the specialness of the couple as a unit of happiness. Stef and Lena, for instance in the first and second season, hover on the verge of dissolution and are haunted by lesbian bed death. In one of the early episodes of the first season, when their lesbian coupled friends are breaking apart, Lena and Stef reflect on their own relationship, focusing especially on their lack of time and drive for sex with each other. As seen in figure 2.1, they take time out of their busy lives to lie down together on their bed and look through schedules on their smartphones to plan a time when they can arrange a sex date. Their failure at sex haunts the edges of their stable family unit, until finally at the end of the episode, they go at it in the car, evaporating the ghost of lesbian bed death that was threatening their coupled structure. In the second season they are less successful, as they both fail to orgasm during sex and "lesbian bed death" gains a presence on the show by formal name this time. As seen in figure 2.2, their unsuccessful sex act results in feeling alienated from each other, awkward, frustrated, and worried about their relationship.

In *The Fosters*, monogamous sex in the context of a long-term partnership holds many promises. It marks the love of the unit, the commitment of each person to the other's pleasure and bodily joy, and an investment in the future of the family upheld by the twin pillars of the couple. As Berlant elucidates, sex is a key organizing ritual of the good life, and when it falls into disrepair in the coupled formation, it causes anxiety as to the survival of the middle-class family unit.[30] Sex functions for Berlant as a practice of "cruel optimism" in that it constitutes an attachment to desires of security, order, and social recognition. A decline in sex, on the other hand, threatens to bring about the attrition of the subject. Sex comes to index, in this way, the good, healthy life, the anchor of family stability in the middle-class context. Stef and Lena succeed at life, as is made evident through their comfortable house, their stable professions, and their capacity to offer love and financial security to their amassed children. Their struggle against lesbian bed death is part of their fight for keeping the good life alive and combating the attrition of the subject that lesbian bed death threatens.

What, then, is the promise of sex? The promise of sex is, first off, an unevenly distributed promise. It serves a biopolitical disciplinary and regulatory function, encouraging normative bodies and populations to maximize their potential for success and health, while barring sex from groups considered harmful, dangerous, or deleterious. The promise is extended along lines of normativity; enforced in white, well-off, and able-bodied populations; and discouraged among racialized, lower-class, precarious groups and people with disabilities. Sex is only happy, healthy, and profound if it is practiced by the "right" people. For those deemed unworthy of the promises of sex, sex does not offer promissory qualities but is discursively figured as death, threat, and danger. For instance, the promise of sex is not often extended to people with disabilities, who are denied sexual pleasure, presumed to not be capable of sex, and banned from sex biopolitically so as to discourage reproduction.[31] Further, the sex that sex workers have is often conceived of as "dangerous" rather than "good" and healthful, pointing to the continued circulation of sex negativity in contemporary contexts. Similarly, until recently, gay sex has been conceived of as not good but lethal, deviant, immoral. As Leo Bersani, Michael Warner, and others have explored, a sex ban was advocated for gay men during the HIV/AIDS "crisis" of the 1980s, channeling homophobia and ableism into the discipline and regulation of gay bodies and communities.[32] Biopolitical at its core, the promise of sex is a relational horizon linked with ideas of whose life is livable and reproducible and with dreams of the optimization of a particular body politic.

The promise of sex is also layered and contradictory in what it offers and who it extends its inviting embrace to. Sex promises health and vitality through a "healthicization of sex" and is exalted as a practice that can optimize, regenerate, and enhance bodily health.[33] In this way, sex is pivoted as a tool for regenerating and maintaining the individual body, the body of the coupled unit, and the body of the population. To be engaged and invested in sex is thus to manifest a healthy body and mind, and to be proactive in thwarting psychological and physiological illness. In this rendition, the promise of sex is the promise of the optimal body, unabridged by illness or disability. Through the optimization of health, the promise of sex is also the promise of the good life fitted with middle-class stature, a coupled relationship unit, a productively happy working life, and community belonging.[34]

Lesbian bed death surfaces as a formation that indexes both the promises of the good life and the fears of its loss. Because, as I have explored, lesbians have traditionally been desexualized through the instrumental usage of its trope, lesbian bed death serves as a feared presence that marks the contours of lesbian identity. Yet the coinage of "lesbian bed death" suggests a conflicted attitude about whether lesbians are indeed worthy of the promises that sex offers, that is, cultural intelligibility, belonging in the body politic, and inclusion in productive capitalist-scapes. In this sense, Stef and Lena's battle against lesbian bed death on ABC's *The Fosters* can also be understood as a navigation of the precarity of lesbian identity and its still fragile inclusion in the citizenship structures of homonationalistic America. Overcoming LBD in mainstreamed lesbian representations is thus tantamount to being able to support, uphold, and celebrate lesbianism in the face of continued homophobic resentment of lesbian love, success, and family living.

To fail at durable, long-term sex in the relational structure of lesbianism presents a multidimensional threat to identity and the promise of sex. In the first case, to fail at sex through lesbian bed death is to capitulate to dominant discursive structures that continue to be skeptical of the possibility of lesbian sex in the first place. In this sense, lesbian bed death, as a lived or representational practice, becomes framed as necessarily bad for lesbianism as an identity. For instance, queer theoretical responses to Lisa Cholodenko's film *The Kids Are All Right* (2010), as Gupta has laid out, flesh out this discomfort and anxiety around representing lesbian bed death.[35] *The Kids Are All Right* follows the white, married lesbian couple Nic (played by Annette Bening) and Jules (played by Julianne Moore) and their two birth children as they navigate the new presence of the children's biological father and their sperm donor, Paul (played by Mark Ruffalo), in their lives. Unlike in *The Fosters* season 1, Nic and Jules, married for many years, are not portrayed as "overcoming" their lesbian bed death despite several attempts to do so. Yet, interestingly, despite the sexlessness of the marriage and Jules's affair with Paul, the marital and family formation survives, providing an account of lesbian marital durability.

Aghast with its representation of lesbianism as sexless, queer theorists such as Jack Halberstam blogged about the ways in which Cholodenko's film representationally fails the identity of lesbianism, since it "loads sexual inertia, domestic dowdiness, and bourgeois complacency onto the lesbian couple" and "seals the moms in asexual pathos."[36] Fascinatingly, as Gupta has discussed in "Picturing Space for Lesbian Nonsexualities" (2013), a large part of the queer dislike for the film is rooted in a rejection of lesbian nonsexualities, a veritable hatred of the trope of lesbian bed death and the sting of failure it carries for the figure of the lesbian couple.[37]

Like in *The Fosters*, *The Kids Are All Right* provides us with a middle-class, coupled, able-bodied, and cisgender representation of lesbianism. The kinship dynamics established in both demonstrate a devotion to the couple and the social institution of the marital couple in particular, which, in the words of Michael Warner, "is designed both to reward those inside it and to discipline those outside it."[38] Unlike *The Fosters*, *The Kids Are All Right* in a sense offers an even more conservative vision of lesbian family making that is caught up in racist whiteness, biological parenthood, heavily gendered marital ideals, and a family unit that protects itself against external breaching. Nic, Jules, their sperm donor Paul, and their children are all stubbornly white, Nic as an OB/GYN is the family's breadwinner while Jules is the stay-at-home mother, and the family ultimately retains its nuclear status through warding off the threat of the sperm donor as an additional parental figure. Even so, unlike in *The Fosters*, Nic and Jules stay together despite their sexlessness and without resolving the trope of lesbian bed death. Thus, unlike in *The Fosters*, *The Kids Are All Right* actually offers a more favorable representation of nonsexuality, which becomes a focal point of detestation for queer critiques of the film. This is not to say that *The Kids Are All Right* is a politically astute film, or to ignore that it has racist tendencies, bourgeois attachments, or an obsession with white subjecthood, but rather, that queer theoretical engagements with

*The Kids Are All Right* are indicative of an almost religious and certainly moral investment in the promises of sex and a chronic anxiety around its breakage.

Of interest here is that the queer fear and dislike of the trope of lesbian bed death is so great that its representation, even in the mainstream, is framed as a failure not only of a single couple but of the lesbian identity itself. Cynthia Barounis, in a compelling asexual analysis of John Cameron Mitchell's *Shortbus* (2006), demonstrates that sexual failure plays a metonymic function, so that an absence of sex speaks not only of the "dysfunctional" or "unliberated" attributes of an individual but also becomes understood as a misrepresentation of an entire identity and a breakage point for an entire imagined community.[39] Since one aspect of the promise of sex is that it "vitalizes and strengthens the bonds of queer and national community," its absence breaks this queer circuit and forsakes the community.[40] The failure of the long-term lesbian couple to have sex thus becomes not only their failure but the failure of lesbianism itself. *The Kids Are All Right* is representationally threatening because it presents lesbianism in proximity to both lesbian bed death and asexuality.

Lesbian bed death, I am arguing, is a threatening cultural formation because it speaks of a threat to the promises of sex. In *The Fosters,* the retaining of sex in the coupled unit provides a continued investment in middle-class family life and inclusion in regimes of productive citizenship. In queer theorists' critiques of *The Kids Are All Right,* we see a discomfort with not only homonormative family structures but also with a lesbian coupling that is nonsexual or that succumbs to lesbian bed death. Yet *The Kids Are All Right* delivers the surprising message that lesbian-based homonormativity can be sustained without sex, vacating sex of some of its promises.

I have been kneading the representational trope of lesbian bed death within mainstreamed lesbian representations with the aim of circling in on cultural, both queer and straight, affixations to sex and its promises. The phraseology, representation, and diagnosis of lesbian bed death is by all means a lesbian-phobic and gendered formation that functions to dismantle lesbian identification. Stemming from stereotypic ideas around lesbian practices, lesbian bed death is also a formation that carries with it homonormative ideals of coupling, whiteness, and middle-class sexuality as well as disciplinary notions of who should be having sex in the first place. Yet in addition to this, lesbian bed death is also a trope that smacks of a hesitancy toward nonsexuality and asexuality, a fear that the dissolution of sex jeopardizes the attributes of identification—in this case, lesbian identification.

To unpack the influential cultural trope of lesbian bed death is thus necessarily to engage in an asexually motivated criticality toward the role of sex in popular representational practices. An asexual reading of lesbian bed death interrogates the need to assert that sex is at the heart of lesbianism. It considers, as I have been doing, the damage this assertion does to those lesbians who are nonsexual in various ways—be it asexually identified, tired and not wanting to have sex, in long-term nonsexual lesbian formations, in "Boston marriages," in lesbian friendships, due to trauma, or who are single or not partaking in sex for a broad host of reasons. In placing asexuality in reference to lesbian bed death, or reading lesbian bed death asexually, I am suggesting that there is a formative proximity between them. Asexual modes of relating arise in lesbian bed death, both as a representational and a lived practice, with fecund possibilities for imagining an asexual erotics.

Arguably, two central projects of lesbian studies have been to beckon lesbianism into visibility, arguing against its invisibilization by mainstream culture, and to demonstrate that lesbianism is sexual, pushing back against its desexualization. These twin goals of lesbian studies are, for instance, visible in Terry Castle's important book *The Apparitional Lesbian* (1993), which, as part of "bring[ing] the lesbian back into focus" asserts that "she [the lesbian] is not asexual."[41] While lesbianism has been defiantly defended as sexual, wherein the sexual is seen as a promissory and sedimenting constituent of the lesbian identity, I ask that we begin to attend to the obvious asexual components of lesbianism.

Lesbian theory and history have in fact had a trajectory of indirect attentiveness to asexuality. As I have been exploring throughout, the work of Audre Lorde formulates a black lesbian erotics that imagines intimacies with other women as exceeding sex and decentering sexual desire.[42] Likewise, Barbara Smith, in "Toward a Black Feminist Criticism" (1977), discussed the power of erotic friendship for black women and girls in a white supremacist patriarchal society that encourages heterosexuality above other relationships. Looking at Toni Morrison's *Sula*, and drawing on the concept of the "woman-identified-woman," she argued that in the novel Sula and Nel share an erotic, deeply sensual relationship that forms the main reference point throughout their lives and must on some level be understood as lesbianism.[43] As the previous chapter explored, asexuality constituted a central erotics in lesbian-feminist organizing in the 1970s and 1980s, as is visible through the figure of the "woman-identified-woman." As articulated by Barbara Smith, Adrienne Rich, and Radicalesbians, lesbian feminism arose as a primarily political orientation, an attraction to women that was motivated not by a lust for sex but by a commitment to building erotic communities, cultures, and friendships with women, oftentimes with revolutionary goals.[44] On the one hand, this evacuated sex from lesbianism, denying the salience of sex and sexual desire to lesbianism and effectively desexualizing lesbians. On the other hand, however, 1970s and 1980s lesbian feminism could be understood as touching on the asexual currents within lesbianism that were later set aside in the fight to ward off stereotypes of lesbian bed death.

Lesbian theory has similarly been indirectly receptive to asexuality through examinations of intimate friendships and expositions of Boston marriages. The work of Lillian Faderman, Martha Vicinus, and Omise'eke Natasha Tinsley each offers explorations of romantic lesbianism that is inclusive of and open to asexual intimacies.[45] For example, Martha Vicinus, in *Intimate Friends* (2004), identified "the openly sexual, to the delicately sensual, to the disembodied ideal" all as "varieties of erotic love."[46] Also, through a rendering of Boston marriages, Faderman, and even more pronouncedly, Esther Rothblum and Kathleen Brehony in *Boston Marriages* (1993), have elaborated on the strong and meaningful aspects of asexuality to lesbianism.[47] As Faderman memorably writes, "'Lesbian' described a relationship in which two women's strongest emotions and affections are directed toward each other. Sexual contact may be a part of the relationship to a greater or lesser degree, or it may be entirely absent."[48] Likewise, Tinsley in her text on Caribbean women writers' decolonizing explorations of women who love women, speaks to eroticism as "a sharing of deep, possibly but not necessarily sexual feeling," articulating lesbianism as about more than sexual desire.[49]

Literature on lesbianism and trauma also provides another way in which asexual modes are central to lesbianism. Leslie Feinberg's *Stone Butch Blues* (1993), which has been taken up as an autobiographical text central to the articulation of both lesbian and transgender identities, provides narratives of an asexuality motivated by the political life of trauma and an unwillingness to touch as central to the embodiment of trauma.[50] While not wanting to be touched cannot be directly mapped onto the sexual identity of asexuality in any obvious way, it does suggest another manner in which nonsexualities are resonant with lesbianism. Further, and as the final section of this chapter will explore, considerations of untouchability and lesbianism also provide a glummer, less celebratory resonance with asexuality, one that does not try to ignore possible histories of trauma and their relationship to both lesbianism and asexuality. Intimate friendship, Boston marriages, the woman-identified-woman, and lesbian trauma can all be fruitfully read as instances of attentiveness to asexual erotics within lesbian studies and indeed as a formative proximity between lesbianism and asexuality.

Conversations to debunk lesbian bed death thus take place against a backdrop of historical and political work that has valued the asexual erotics of lesbian identification. I am not suggesting that lesbianism is or should be asexual but rather that there is fecund proximity and overlap between the twin iden-tifications of asexuality and lesbianism that can easily be discounted when the focus remains on proving that lesbians are sexual. More broadly, I am also suggesting that in order to fully study lesbian identity, representation, and the figure of the bed, we need to release our hold on the sexual as the default mode of relationality, attending to asexually erotic forms of relating. Asexuality is a crucial component of relationality and a possible ground for erotic and queer articulations of being with others and being with oneself. An attentiveness to asexuality is integral to the study of sexuality, queerness, and lesbianism.

## BED: THE BED IN LESBIAN ART

To trace the asexual resonances of lesbian bed death, I will now unpack one of the key coordinating elements of lesbian bed death's phraseology: namely, the bed. The bed is a key site for an analysis of lesbian bed death not only because it becomes the living memorial for the anxiety of sex's failure but also because it can be read as indexing lesbian potentiality for asexuality. In turning to the bed as a figure central in lesbian art, I hope to read the bed asexually, expand-ing the archive of asexual figures, tropes, representations, and moments. By referring to "lesbian art," I have in mind a genre of art that is created either by or for communities of lesbian-identified folk of various genders that touches on topics, desires, and politics of relevance to lesbianism.[51] In distinction to the mainstreamed representations of lesbianism explored in the previous sec-tion, lesbian art tends to speak to communities that are more deeply invested in questions of lesbianism and more attuned to the shifting debates and poli-tics within. In other words, lesbian art is countercultural art directed at queer, lesbian, and feminist counterpublics and goes against the social norms and taken-for-granted ideas of the mainstream.[52] As such, lesbian art is distinct from mainstreamed representations of lesbianism.

The bed has long played a pivotal role in both art and lesbian art. We can think of the lineage of the bed in art as spanning Frida Kahlo's bed paintings and bed-based painting practice, Robert Rauschenberg's canonized *Bed* (1955) and Tracey Emin's *My Bed* (1998), Félix González-Torres's empty beds (1991) featured on New York's billboards as a response to the AIDS epidemic, Yoko Ono and John Lennon's bed-in during their honeymoon in 1969 at the Hilton Hotel in Amsterdam in response to the Vietnam War, Diane Arbus's photo-graph *Two Friends at Home, N. Y. C.* (1965), and more recently the activist art project by student Emma Sulkowicz, who after not having her sexual assault taken seriously by Columbia University, took to carrying her mattress around with her on campus in the endurance piece *Mattress Performance* (2015).[53] Notably, the bed, while referential of our most private moments—sleep, rest, pain, death, sex—has been a politically astute symbol in feminist and queer art especially. It often provides a comment on the refusal to keep trauma hidden behind four walls, making arguments for the politically and socially relevant content of what would otherwise be understood as personal misfortune. Featuring the bed in artwork has functioned for artists as a challenge to the domestic containment, invisibility, and depoliticization of illness, disability, sexual assault, trauma, and homophobia. Kahlo's paintings affectively map out her experiences with disability, Rauschenberg's *Bed* (1955) is remembered for speaking to his gay identity, Emin's *My Bed* (1998) is a refusal to keep femininity contained and sanitized, González-Torres's billboards (1991) hold society responsible for homophobia and the mistreatment of people with HIV/AIDS, and Sulkowicz's *Mattress Performance* (2015) holds her rapist and university publically accountable while bringing sexual trauma into the public sphere.

The bed, in short, is intimately entangled with not only sex but also a host of other life events and day-to-day practices as well as their political contexts. It serves as a symbolic site through which to navigate questions of identity and trauma. The two bed series I will consider, Tammy Rae Carland's *Lesbian Beds* (2002) and *Lesbian Bedrooms II* (2011) by Kyle Lasky, adapt the focus on the bed in art to think through questions of lesbian identity as they pertain to visibility, desexualization, and the category of "lesbianism" itself. They both, in different and overlapping ways, provide a narrative of lesbian entanglement with the bed, an entanglement that is both sexual and asexual at once.

Tammy Rae Carland's *Lesbian Beds* from 2002, speaking directly against claims to lesbian bed death, is a series of thirteen full-color aerial photos of beds left in disarray after their inhabitants have departed for the day (see figure 2.3).[54] Carland indicates that they draw on modernist styles and are referential in particular of Rauschenberg's canonized piece *Bed* (1955), a combine of pillow, quilt, and sheets covered with oil paint, hung on the wall like a painting.[55] While Rauschenberg's *Bed* (1955) is commonly said to speak to his love affair with equally canonized artist Jasper Johns, it has an asexual node, since as a single, abandoned bed "it is unclear . . . whether this particular bed points to the renunciation of sex or its exhibition."[56] Kenneth Silver argues that it can be read both asexually and sexually, since it speaks to a "monk's asceticism" as a form of devotion to art making while also being potentially suggestive of the "sexual writhings appearing indexically in the wild paint splattered."[57] This ambiguity over the sexualness of Rauschenberg's *Bed* points to the ways in which beds can be polyvocal erotic symbols of a/sexual expression and identity.

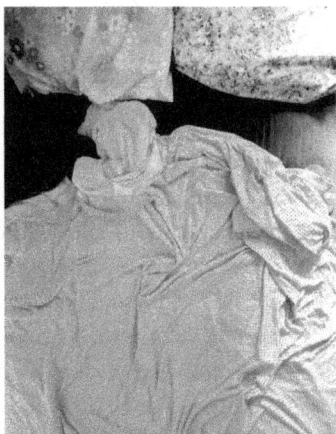

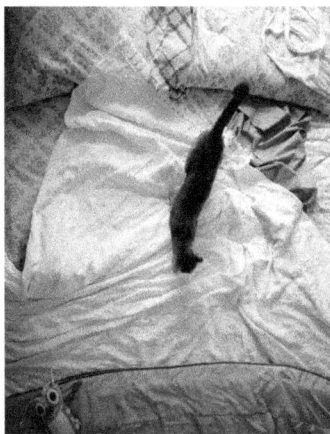

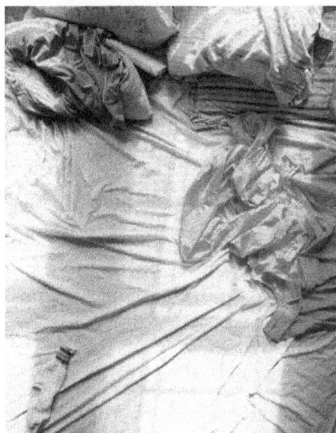

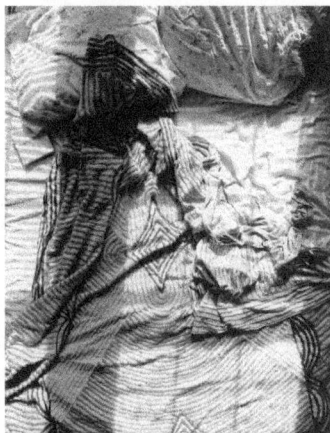

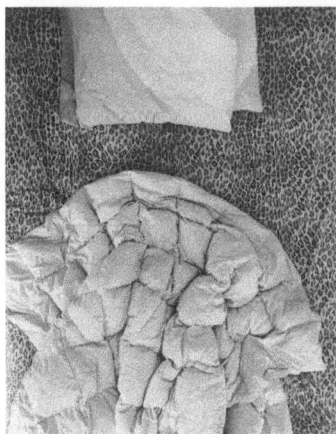

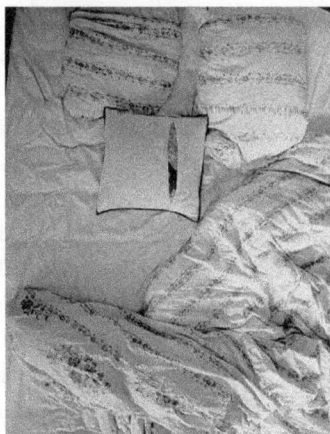

**FIGURE 2.3.** Tammy Rae Carland, *Lesbian Beds,* 2002. Reprinted with permission of Tammy Rae Carland. Copyright the artist. Courtesy the artist and Jessica Silverman Gallery, San Francisco, with grateful acknowledgment to Beryl Bevilacque from the gallery.

*Lesbian Beds* (2002) also draws on a history of feminist art making, which likewise focalized the bed as a site of interrogating gendered public and private lifescapes. Specifically, Emin's art installation *My Bed* (1998), featured in the Saatchi Gallery, was of an unmade bed covered in the detritus of daily life during her "complete absolute breakdown."[58] It featured the unrest and unwellness characterizing her life and was marked by cigarette butts, alcohol bottles, used stockings, condoms, a used tampon, and contraceptive pills.[59] Referencing Rauschenberg explicitly and Emin's work implicitly, Carland's *Lesbian Beds* speaks against both the invisibility of lesbianism and its desexualization, seeking to, in Carland's own words, "reinsert a non-heteronormative women's sexuality into and onto photographic discourse, art history and domestic sites of pleasure and intimacy."[60] Creating a symbology that is not heteronormatively bound, Carland's work puts forward the bed as a site of erotic investment for lesbian intimacy.

Similarly, *Lesbian Bedrooms II* (2011) by Kyle Lasky provides a full-color photographic archive of lesbians in situ in their bedrooms (see figure 2.4). Lesbianism here is deliberately expanded to broaden understandings of who might "count" or "pass" under its identity.[61] Lasky undertook the series as a male and trans-masculine person with continued investments in lesbian communities and butch lesbianism and with an interest in complexifying lesbian identity. Lasky's photographs challenge biologically determinist understandings of lesbianism and dismantle lesbianism's investment in a gender binary. The goal for Lasky is thus not merely to "normalize the intimacy that passed between lesbians" in the sense of speaking against both their invisibilization and desexualization, but also to combat "a traditional notion of lesbian identity . . . so rooted in this idea of 'women-born-women-loving-women.'"[62] The series both celebrates and reworks lesbian identification, suggesting, as Lasky frames it, that "lesbian identity is not so much a sexual orientation, but a political orientation" drawn out of a history of feminist work and antisexist and antihomophobic cultures.[63] Lesbianism emerges as something that is less about the gender of one's object choice and sexual orientation than about the networks, communities, and friendships one forms, and how one is formed by these. In *Lesbian Bedrooms II* the bed emerges as a key platform for expanding the possibilities of lesbian erotics and identity and navigating community.

Carland's and Lasky's photographic series share many formal elements in common. Not only do they both make use of the bed as a referent for lesbianism, they also both consist of carefully composed and contained tableaus, animated by objects, fabrics, textures, and colors. Both Carland and Lasky complicate the clarity and expand the visuality of the category of "lesbianism"—Lasky through a deliberate inclusion of varying queer embodiments

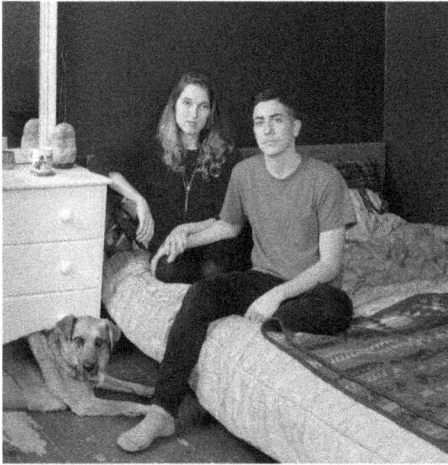

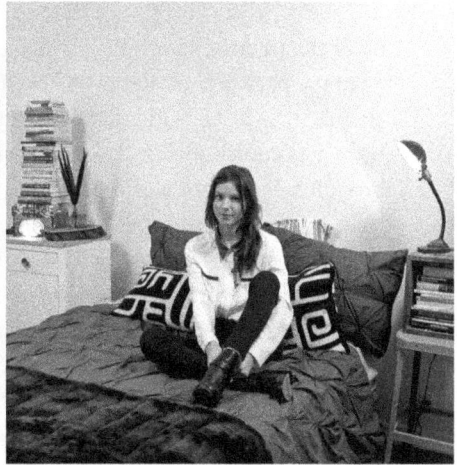

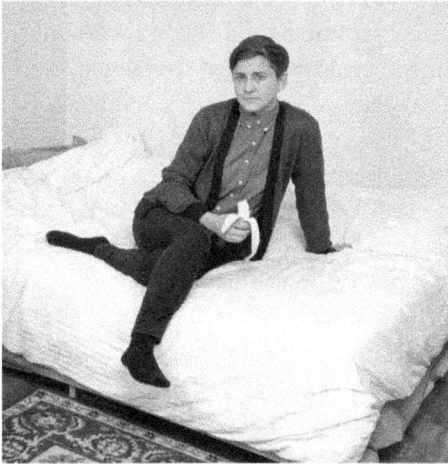

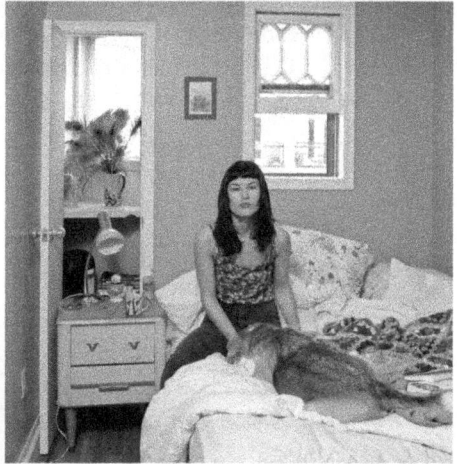

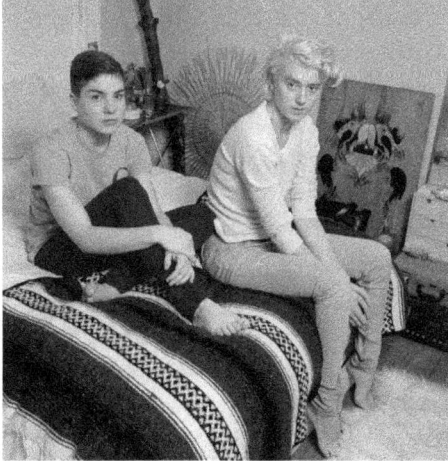

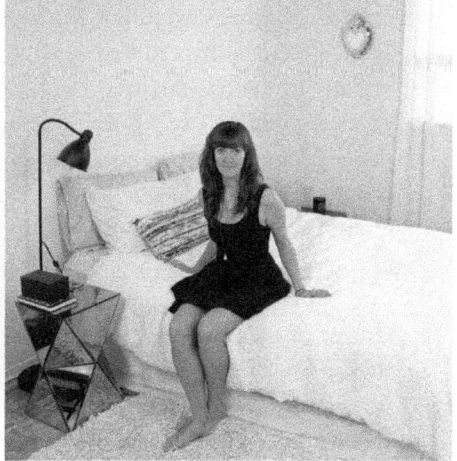

**FIGURE 2.4.** Kyle Lasky, *Lesbian Bedrooms II,* 2011. Copyright and courtesy of the artist.

under the politicized terrain of "the lesbian," and Carland through an absenting of the person from her beds, leaving us to guess who the beds' lesbians are, complicating lesbian identity (who gets to count as a "lesbian") and practice (what acts constitute lesbianism). Both series also form a sense of community through a consistent and repeating framing of the bed and bedroom, respectively, that creates linkages and connections between lesbians and their beds.

Both Carland's and Lasky's photographs balance a deliberation between lesbianism as both private and public, sexual and asexual, formulating an ambiguous lesbian erotics. Engaging with the trope of lesbian bed death, they both respond to the desexualization of lesbianism through situating it squarely at the site of domesticity and bedroom intimacy. In *Lesbianism, Cinema, Space: The Sexual Life of Apartments* (2009), Lee Wallace argues that while lesbianism used to be representationally situated in the narrative space of the bar, the schoolroom, the prison, and the college, the second half of the twentieth century saw the shift to the apartment "as the privileged spatial marker of lesbian possibility."[64] The apartment straddles personal privacy and public engagement, serving also as a marker of lesbian domesticity and as a "sexual space."[65] While queer theory has tended to overprioritize public sex as a site of transgression and domestic sex as a repository of conservative intimacy, representational practices such as Carland's and Lasky's photo series reference lesbianism through the domestic space.[66] Wallace argues that enshrining lesbianism in domestic spaces "risks [it] being considered asexual," and I would like to agree: Carland's and Lasky's photographs, while ardently working to disprove lesbian bed death, actually also reference lesbian bed death, as well as the ambivalent asexual resonances within lesbianism.[67]

Further, Carland's and Lasky's photographs are potent with asexual erotics. As I have been exploring, the beds in Carland's and Lasky's series function both as a celebration and as a memorial to sex. On the one hand, they speak visually to the desexualization of lesbianism and try to combat lesbian bed death through an explicit link between the bed and the lesbian. For Carland, the bed in its dynamic unmadeness references perhaps a sex act (or sleep act) completed, speaking with vibrancy and texture to the erotic quality of lesbian quotidian life. Carland's beds are suggestive of erotic worlds left behind when one exits the bed. They are brightly lit, as a bed might be upon morning rising, and contain a light celebration of lesbian erotics. While mostly featuring tangles of pillows, blankets, and duvets, there are also other signs of life: a sock, a cat, a book, a stuffed animal.

In Lasky's *Lesbian Bedrooms II* (2011), the photographs' subjects, in either solitary or coupled formations, sit or lie on the bed, looking solemnly at the viewer while resting on mostly neatly made beds in well-organized bedrooms.

With solemn facial expressions and relaxed body postures, the photos' subjects look back at the viewer who might want to intrusively enter their space. While nonhuman friends and couples are included in the series, many of the photographs feature solitary subjects. At the same time, community is implied through the consistent framing of the bedrooms, suggesting continuity between bedrooms, a lesbian erotics that connects lesbians to each other across their homes.

Dana Seitler, in her exploration of Carland's *Lesbian Beds* (2002), asks, "Can aesthetics be queer?" and this similar question can also be posed in regard to asexuality: Can aesthetics be asexual, or perhaps more to the point, what is asexual in Carland's and Lasky's photographs?[68] First, *Lesbian Beds* (2002) offers a celebration of lesbian eroticism that is not strictly sexual, in that the images are not strictly about sex or sexual desire. Because the lesbian referent is absent, we are left to infer what the bed offers in each of these photos—and the answer is not self-evidently sexual. While colorful and textured, the beds are also abandoned, vacated, posited as a memorial to sex, or at least the residue of a night. There is a mark of loss and departure on the beds. The asexual resonance of these photographs lies in their ambivalence around sex, their indeterminacy as to what role sex plays in regard to the bed, and their deferral of an explicit link between bodies-at-sex and the bed.

In Lasky's *Lesbian Bedrooms II* (2011), asexuality, and arguably aromantic asexuality, takes on a formal element. While peopled, these photographs, like Carland's, for the most part do not contain explicit sexual content. Even more so, in most cases the subjects are cool and collected, alone or, if coupled, barely touching. Yet the photos are highly erotic. In one, the subject holds a bitten banana; in another, a dog's face is obscured as its attention is channeled toward the person. In all the photos, the subjects stare coolly and confidently at the camera, the photographer, and the viewer. I read the photographs as charged with an eroticism that is in part asexual, an invitation not to touch necessarily, but to occupy a zone of lesbian identification that is pliable, that is unconstricted, and that tingles across time and context. I read the photographs as an invitation to capacious lesbianism, one that is both inclusive of asexuality and charged with eroticism.

While Carland's series is perhaps more easily read as a celebration of sex in its unkempt and dynamic rendition of the bed, suggestive of a site on which some event took place (be it sleep, or sex, or otherwise), neither series is strictly about sex or about demonstrating that lesbians need sex as part of their erotic practice. Even compared to Emin's *My Bed* (1998), which centralized bodily fluids and carnal urges through the presence of condoms, tampons, and contraceptive pills, Lasky's and Carland's series are by comparison fairly sanitized, exempt of sex toys or explicitly sexual content. In this sense, both series obliquely reference a certain relation to sex that is fueled by the continued presence of lesbian bed death.

Also, both series draw on the genre of lesbian art and reference a sense of community and erotics found among lesbians and queers even as they do not include signs and symbols that are usually held as representative of "community," such as holding hands, embracing, or being clustered in groups. The sense of community rests instead on the consistent and repeating composition sequence of each series and the erotic conversation formed between the photographs and the viewer. In the consistent framing of the beds and bedrooms, respectively, a lesbian erotics takes shape that connects lesbians to each other across their homes. This erotics is markedly not only about sexual desire but also an erotic longing for community that is in part asexual. Even while beds are so central to both series, both artists implicitly reference lesbian bed death without passing any judgment on the level of sexual desire or sex within each lesbian bed. With a hesitant rejection of lesbian bed death as a representational trope and practice, both series, in unique ways, are resonant with the asexual content and erotics of lesbian day-to-day life. While perhaps rejecting lesbian bed death, neither *Lesbian Bedrooms II* (2011) nor *Lesbian Beds* (2002) draws on the pernicious implications for asexuality that queer critiques of LBD usually imply, such as that to not have sex or desire sex is to be a failed lesbian or to do damage to the queer community as a whole.[69] The lesbian communities in both series, and especially in Lasky's, survive and flourish despite no clear indication of sex or sexual desire or even of "coming together." Instead a deeper, broader, more gender-inclusive, and asexually inclusive erotics is formulated visually—one that is neither compulsively happy nor compulsively sexual.

## DEATH: ASEXUAL EROTICS OF FAILURE

It could be said that lesbian bed death offers us an unoptimistic form of asexuality. This is not to say that lesbian bed death cannot be a site of joy and intimacy formation in the context of a long-term lesbian couple, but rather that the trope itself is connotative of failure and glumness. Lesbian bed death, as a three-word formation, is not only caught up in pernicious accounts of lesbian identity but it also binds lesbianism to death. It renders both lesbianism and asexual resonances of sexual absence as sites of loss, death, and failure. In this way, LBD forms a moribund relationality that, as I have been exploring, has been framed as doing damage to lesbianism, and further, has the potential to do symbolic harm to the optimistic qualities of pride-based asexuality movements. In this final section, I explore LBD as an erotics of failure.

In my work, I get asked so often to validate asexuality as a real sexual orientation by "proving" that asexuals face discrimination. Pride-based approaches have become such a strong tool of LGBTQ2+ movements because of this expectation that marginalized sexual and gender identities are all about suffering and pain (and putting the pain on display for straight and cisgender publics). In relation to asexuality, to not be harassed and discriminated against is thus tantamount to not existing as a sexual orientation or identity in the first place. When I am asked to "prove" asexual discrimination, I am invited to disprove asexuality as a legitimate sexual identity. As I outlined in the introduction, while "asexuals as a group are not perceived as being specifically targeted by institutionally oppressive forces," there is mounting evidence that asexuals experience both implicit and explicit discrimination.[70] In a cultural context that privileges sex and sexual desire and undermines nonsexualities, asexuality becomes a deposit site for pernicious connotations that are visible as well in the trope of lesbian bed death.

To combat the perceived glumness of the asexual subject by the mainstream, asexual activists have embraced optimistic approaches to sharing knowledge and experiences of asexuality, proving that asexuality exists through a different set of tactics than calling on discrimination. Because asexuals have been routinely represented by popular media as sad, dejected, lacking losers, asexual visibility politics are often committed to profiling a happy, "normal," healthful asexuality. Representations of asexuality as a healthy, happy state that does not impede on compulsory sexuality or challenge social structures also function to gain currency for asexuality by providing a nonthreatening image of the identity. Asexuality's validity is argued through a logic that asexuals are "normal" and that asexuality is not coterminous with trauma, depression, or experiences of sexual assault. An overemphasis on happiness in public renditions of asexuality is a strategy for staving off negative stereotypes, but, like with other sexual identities, it can all too readily rely on ableist liberal reassurances of health and happiness. Pride-full representations can cut asexuality off from disability, trauma, and pain with the hope of asserting the "normalcy" of asexuality as a sexual identity among sexual identities.[71] This positive approach to asexual visibility also puts pressure on people who are asexual to be happy ambassadors for asexuality, pushing a liberal agenda of normality, success, and life fulfillment for the good of identity recognition.

In turn, exploring asexual resonances that are rendered representationally glum provides an interesting counterpoint to this emphasis on a happy, healthy image of asexuality and its participation in the upkeep of sex and its promises. Lesbian bed death homes in on the darker connotations of asexuality that associate a perceived lack of sex or sexual desire with failure on various fronts: the loss of productivity, ill health, absence of intimacy, unhappiness, waning of vitality, and attrition of the subject. It challenges not only the presumed universality of sex within lesbianism but also the presumed happiness of asexuality. Considering these darker affective modes of asexual representation, such as LBD, can thus in itself be the ground for the development of an asexual reading that pries apart our investments in the uneven distributions of the promises of sex.

Having examined lesbian bed death throughout this chapter, I wish to suggest that I have been undertaking this analysis through a glum affective stance—an "asexuality without optimism." Berlant's and Edelman's formulation of "sex without optimism" seeks to explore, in part, the anxiety and strangeness of sex, being curious about sex while skeptical of "the sort of sexual optimism implicit in sexual liberation."[72] Heteronormativity, as they explore, has a way of framing "libidinal unruliness" through negative formulations of shame and pathology, eliciting in LGBTQ2+ subjects a commitment to visibility and optimism as a means to combat this dark framing and erasure.[73] Homonormativity is also imbued with an imperative that gay people be happy in that they should both "embrace who they are" and be grateful to the powers that be for their supposed inclusion in the fabric of life.[74] As Heather Love has written of "compulsory happiness":

> In the era of gay normalisation, gays and lesbians not only have to be like everybody else . . . they have to look and feel good doing it. . . . For gay Americans, the pressure to appear in good spirits is even greater. Because homosexuality is traditionally so closely associated with disappointment and depression, being happy signifies participation in the coming era of gay possibility.[75]

Homonormativity is further harnessed by the state as a racist tool useful in justifying American exceptionalism, invasion, and the disposal of racialized bodies.[76] In this sense, "queer" is evacuated of political context also in that it comes to serve white supremacist and nationalist ends—that is, in the words of David Eng, "queer liberalism" serves a "narrowly pragmatic gay and lesbian identity and identity politics, the economic interests of neoliberalism and whiteness, and liberal political norms of inclusion."[77] While asserting happiness as a sexual or gender minority is in itself a powerful act against erasure and pathologization, happiness is all too easily harnessed by capitalism.

Challenging tropes of the happily assimilated LGBT subject, queer and lesbian studies have provided effective modes of thinking about trauma and nonoptimistic or negative affects. Ann Cvetkovich, in *An Archive of Feelings* (2003), directly examined the entwinement of trauma with lesbianism, presenting an affective challenge to the happy imperative that strives to make minoritarian cultures and identities more palatable to society through "assimilation, inclusion, and normalcy."[78] In different ways, Sara Ahmed and Jack Halberstam have theorized the killjoy and failure, respectively, as oppositional affects that refuse to abide by a happy imperative that uses happiness instrumentally toward the maintenance of unjust social orders.[79] Drawing on these texts and on Berlant and Edelman, "asexuality without optimism" similarly refuses to utilize asexuality only through homonormative, homonationalist, and homocelebratory language. While ace pride is as important a project as other pride movements in that it builds community, carves out spaces of legibility, and generates new modes of being, I offer "asexuality without optimism" as a twin strategy for reading asexual resonances, and one that is effective at thinking about an erotics of failure such as the moniker of lesbian bed death presents. "Asexuality without optimism"—what I have engaged in throughout this chapter—traces the darker affective undercurrents of sexual lack, low levels of sexual desire, and forms of nonsexuality articulated in popular parlance as "failure" or failed sexuality. Failure, Halberstam has explored, is integral to queer temporalities that thwart restrictive norms and celebrate the successes of adulthood along heteronormative lines. It is accompanied by "a host of negative affects, such as disappointment, disillusionment, and despair" while "pok[ing] holes in the toxic positivity of contemporary life."[80] Ironically, while Halberstam is all about failure, he was, as I have explored, uninterested in seeing lesbian bed death or lesbian sexual lack as a provocative embodiment of failure that directs us to poke holes in the promises of sex as it adheres to positivity and homonormative identity maintenance. Drawing on queer formulations of failure, "asexuality without optimism" ponders what erotic forms are left unexamined in a quest for recognizing the happy and celebratory aspects of sexual identity. In regard to lesbianism, I have been arguing that low sexual frequency and low sexual desire have been wrapped up in the derisive parlance of lesbian bed death to legitimize lesbianism and include it in happy citizenship models that rely on sex for stability.

## TOWARD ASEXUALLY EROTIC LESBIANISM

Examining lesbian bed death, I have been interested in reading asexually against pride-based celebrations of asexuality and sexual celebrations of lesbianism. Instead, I have been exploring how sex for lesbianism has been politically and representationally tied to the success of the couple and identity in contexts of compulsory sexuality. If certain forms of sex, lesbian sex included, can serve as stories of love and more importantly "success," lesbian bed death stands in as an asexual erotics of failure. An erotics of failure in this sense relies on a disavowal of celebratory rhetoric in relation to identity formation, and an attunement to the darker modes of queerness.[81] This chapter has argued for the importance of rereading lesbian bed death from an asexual stance. It has followed the concept of lesbian bed death through clinical literature's attachment of lesbianism to sexual failure, mainstream representations of LBD in *The Fosters* and *The Kids Are All Right*, and lesbian art's asexual erotics in Kyle Lasky's *Lesbian Bedrooms II* (2011) and Tammy Rae Carland's *Lesbian Beds* (2002). A turn to asexuality does not require turning our back on sexual practices and identities, but rather encourages a study of the disciplinary and regulatory structures of sex—that is, a commitment to unpacking sex's promises. Thus, a key goal for this chapter has been to identify asexuality as an ignored but persistent tenet in lesbianism, and one that can furnish a fruitful critique of sex that might shift the weight of "lesbian bed death" from a pernicious idiom to an asexual erotic practice.

# CHAPTER 3

# Growing into Asexuality

## *The Queer Erotics of Childhood*

## ON FAMILIAL PLEASURES

During a family visit several years ago, my mother found me affectionately joking with my niece, whose pants, a size too large, I caught slipping down her waist to reveal a child's exposed bum. After much family deliberation about what her fellow schoolchildren would think at seeing her butt so exposed and how a better-fitting pair of pants was required, I joked lovingly about how the other schoolchildren might assume they saw the moon rising in the sky. Amidst love play from the family—my niece, her mother, her grandmother, and me—my mother remarked that she found my comment alarming, presumably on account that, because it came from a queer aunt, it itself was deviant, inflicting deviancy, perversion, or sexualization on my niece. Quickly blown over with further play and affectionate pant-struggle (as my niece's jeans continued to slide down her legs along with her underwear), my mother's rebuff pricked me in how it got at that uncomfortable tangle around sexuality, queerness, and childhood.

Two competing views emerge to speak on behalf of the child's sexuality. The first is the insistence on the child's right to sexual purity, sexual innocence. The right, in other words, for my niece, as a child, to be protected from the purportedly lewd gaze of her ambiguously loving aunt. This right cuts in many ways, editing eroticism out of familial tangles, touches, nudities while also inflicting bad feelings on the participants of intimate moments, disciplining naked bums. In this account, the bum, the crotch, the little niplets, what have you, must be removed from lewd gazes, including those of queer aunties or maybe even touchy-feely grandmothers. Crucially, the protective stance that seeks to preserve sexual purity and innocence by carving off a space unsullied by sexuality is also a racialized stance, as it is frequently a white childhood that is being saved from lascivious gazes, since, in the words of sexual education scholar Jessica Fields, "childhood sexual innocence [is] a notion imbued with racial and gender stereotypes that rely on and reinforce social inequalities."[1] It is also, as my mother's anxiety around the proximity of my queerness to a child's body suggests, fueled by a homophobic coupling of sexual predatoriness with queerness—that is, by what Gayle Rubin identified as the "domino theory of sexual peril," which is convinced that gayness breeds pedophilia.[2]

The second view, a critique of children's desexualization, insists instead on the child's right to sexual agency, sexual subjecthood. In this account, my sweet and bratty niece is sexually desiring, and rightfully so, and even more so, being part of a family network—mothers, grandmothers, aunts—involves an erotic energy that is, and must be, sexual. So what if the bum becomes a site of the child's pleasure? So what if the pleasure of touching spurred by jeans sliding is felt intergenerationally, including by the child and her queer auntie? Queer theory, in particular, has encouraged us to think critically about why the child is sanitized and desexualized in particular ways, while calling into question the division between the categories of "childhood" and "adulthood." It challenges the assumption that this space I occupy, purportedly of "adulthood" (or queer aunthood), is sexual, while the space of another enfleshed being, under the sign of "child," is not.

In the previous two chapters, I explored feminist organizing and lesbian representation, respectively, for their asexual erotics. In this chapter, I continue in the spirit of the previous chapters to explore the ways in which queer theory is informed by asexuality and the ways it disarticulates itself from asexuality. I think on the broad terrain of intergenerational love toward better understanding the asexual erotics of intimate loving, including in the face of trauma.

This chapter is divided in two and animated by several sections. In the first half, I undertake a consideration of how children are desexualized within American contexts as well as recuperated as sexual by queer theory. In the bottom half of the chapter, I undertake a few readings of intergenerational erotics toward better understanding the asexual aspects of familial intimacies. I explore whether it is possible to envision erotic childhood and intergenerational desires without succumbing to a sexual presumption that elides, force-fully or neglectfully, possibilities for asexual development. I do this by first reading Maggie Nelson's recent "auto-theoretical" tract on maternity, child-hood, queerness, identity, and desire, *The Argonauts* (2015), from an asexually attuned standpoint.[3] In reading Nelson, I place her in conversation with Val-erie Solanas and postulate that one way of theorizing asexuality and asexual temporality is by seeing it as something one grows *into* rather than out of, as it is more commonly framed.[4] In the final section, I turn to several pieces of queer art devoted to intergenerational loving, Catherine Opie's iconic work on mothering/parenting (1993 and 2004) and Vivek Shraya's engagement with daughterhood in *Trisha* (2016).[5] In reading this art, I explore questions of whiteness as a racialized standpoint that enables childhood and motherhood to be articulated as "innocent" and, drawing on José Esteban Muñoz, as an affective performance that diminishes other forms of being in the world.[6] I put forward another form of asexual temporality I frame as "time spells," which is evident in the traumatic time travel of both Opie's and Shraya's work and which helps to describe the ambiguous—both sexual and asexual—nature of intergenerational love and longing. By framing sexual and asexual as separate, I am not suggesting that asexuality is not a sexual identity or that it does not fall under the regime of sexuality, but rather that asexual modes of erotics are not underscored by sexual desire in the way that sexual modes of erotics are. Indeed, one aspect of what makes both artists' work so evocative is their abil-ity to queer and to trouble the tales woven about childhood and parenting, such as those of children's sexual "innocence," adult "sexual" desire, or the pastness of parenting and being parented, creating different articulations of the temporalities of intergenerational erotics. Donning the specs of the queer auntie, this chapter studies intergenerational relating not with the loving care of the parental viewer, but with the playful air of someone who wants to do mischief to the sexual longings of children and adults alike.

## KEEPING SEXUALITY UNDER THE BELT

Following the scene of family nudity I depicted, my niece has taken, either through enforcement from her mother or grandmother (or most likely, both), to wearing a big belt to hold her pants securely in place. The belt, which con-tinues to fail to hold up her pants, serves as a potent chastity belt symbol for familial attempts of keeping sexuality hidden, locked away, tucked in deep into the pant legs. In what follows, I will narrativize the desexualization of children by looking at how ideas of asexuality as "arrested" development and childhood as sexually "innocent" are both predicated on racist and ableist temporalities. Next I provide an account of queer and other attempts at unfastening the belt of desexualization, and follow this finally with some initial thoughts as to where this might leave asexuality.

Childhood asexuality is often rendered impossible within queer theory because it smacks of the repression of desexualization. Asexuality is rendered, at best, irrelevant and unnecessary to queer analysis, and at worst, bad politically, functioning to undercut sex and sexuality's centralizing energy in queer community and politics. Michael Warner writes in *The Trouble with Normal* (1999) that "it is inhumane to mandate asexual life for anyone, let alone for queers, for whom sexual culture is a principal mode of sociability and public world making."[7] Writing on HIV/AIDS, Warner rightfully recognizes the harms of desexualizing gay men as a form of social regulation and homophobia. Yet Warner does not articulate how the mandating of sexual desire for queerness and queer identification likewise plays a constraining role. As I explored in the previous chapter, Cynthia Barounis has argued that sex and sexual desire are so key to the "queer utopian project" that "sexual culture [is imagined] as *the* key to solidifying the bonds of queer community."[8] In this sense, sex and sexual desire become prescribed, including at the expense of asexualities.

Asexuality is frequently framed as a marker of immaturity, closetedness, presexuality, or stunted development. As asexuality studies scholar and creative writer M. Milks discusses:

> Asexuality is constructed as an immature, underdeveloped, and incomplete form of pre-sexuality suffering from stunted growth. After all, sexual liberation is ultimately a maturity narrative, a progress myth moving toward an endpoint of total sexual agency that is both individualized and linked to a vision of social transformation; and sexual politics serves a pedagogical, almost messianic role in shepherding its disciples toward this future of transcendent autonomy.[9]

Notions of "stunted" or "arrested" development are entwined with ideas of racial superiority and eugenicist intentions. Jake Pyne explores how "arrested development" evolved as a concept through the ableist idea of "mental deficiency" in the nineteenth century and was used to enforce desexualization through the sterilization and institutionalization of poor people, Indigenous people, people of color, gay people, and people with disabilities.[10] The time scapes of "deficiency" and "arrest" arose in the context of Darwinian understandings of reproduction of the fit and colonial understandings of the

Great Chain of Being, where arrest was used to describe people of color as "trapped" in time while marking whiteness as the culmination of forward-moving human progress.[11] The term "arrested development" also appears in Freud's work when discussing so-called deviant sexualities such as asexual people arrested in their sexual development or gay people arrested in their heterosexual development, yet it does not shed its references to ableism or white supremacy. Asexuality's usage as a form of backwardness, stunted or arrested development, must thus be understood as also drawing on these temporal models of progress and their attachments to whiteness and ability. That people who are asexual past the realm of childhood are figured as developmentally behind or underdeveloped, and rendered as incommensurable with queerness, speaks to investments in particular models of temporal development and lasting notions of superiority, fitness, and ability.

When queerness is edited out of childhood, such as through the temporal framework of "arrest," it is edited out in all its many forms, including asexuality. School curricula, for instance, edit out not only gayness and nonbinary gender and transgender development but also asexual development. As society is not widely familiar with asexuality, it is not seen as a necessary component of a sexual education curriculum. Ironically, even while childhood is desexualized, and sexual education tends to erase sexuality out of curricula, there is a hidden curriculum, which takes for granted that children will transform into sexual adults. Expectations that adults will grow into being sexual—that is, grow into being interested in sex and propelled by sexual desire—are grounded in ideas about the naturalness of sexuality and reproduction as emblems of a fit, able, and willing white citizenry. In other words, the "straightening effects" that take place in childhood and youth are entangled in a developmental narrative that sees sexuality as its end goal, even while sanitizing sexual expression along the way.[12]

There is persistent slippage in queer and nonqueer work alike between the terms "asexuality" and "desexualization" in that both come to, unfortuitously, mean one and the same. In other words, until very recently, asexuality has stood in for desexualization and has rarely been articulated as a positive site of identity or sexual expression. Instead, being subsumed into the negative force of desexualization, asexuality comes to signal a sexuality taken away, a sexuality denied, a sexuality forbidden. Yet, asexuality is not an elaboration of something lost or denied; it is, quite conversely, a marker of something found and understood about oneself, a site of self-meaning, a welcome term in the process of self-understanding. Relying on models of asexuality as a "stunting" or "arrest" rests on ideas entangled in whiteness and ability that ground proper development as necessitating sex. In regard to children, desexualization can include a censorship of sexual knowledge from children, corporeal punishment for being caught with one's hand in one's pants, or the general representational and ideological horizon that Rubin frames as "sex negativity," which convinces children of the morally corrupt nature of sex and sexuality. The insistence on children's "sexual purity" hinges on a devotion to seeing the child as existing in a state that cannot be sexually desiring, driven by the conviction that this would tarnish childhood and its "innocence."

This narrative of childhood innocence is a racial position, and as Fields examines, while children's sexual innocence might be formulated generically, it has a racialized history linked to whiteness in the US.[13] White childhood is preserved through an attachment to desexualization, and yet this "powerful western image of childhood innocence," Dorothy Roberts holds, "does not seem to benefit Black [and racialized] children [who are] born guilty."[14] Black children have historically, in US and Canadian contexts in particular, not been entitled to notions of childhood innocence because they existed as property rather than as "children" under slavery.[15] Notably, these notions around childhood continue to live with us as a legacy of slavery such that white and black children of the same age are portrayed differentially by the media: white children as innocent, and black children as little adults rather than as children. Segregation, in turn, has functioned to protect white children, perceived as innocent, from black children, perceived as guilty, suspect, and endowed with criminality. These discourses and legacies of childhood innocence are reliant also on discourses of "racial innocence" that are invested in the continuing project of rendering white people free of moral blame while generating rhetoric that criminalizes and holds suspect bodies of color.[16] Journalist Ta-Nehisi Coates has called this "the politics of exoneration," in which white people strive to render themselves free of the moral blame for racism.[17] Along similar lines, Eve Tuck and K. Wayne Yang, in relation to settler colonialism, have described "moves to innocence," which "problematically attempt to reconcile settler guilt and complicity, and rescue settler futurity."[18] In both these senses, whiteness itself is held to be a childish state of innocence and naivety, as well as a site of robust maturity and evolutionary superiority all at once. Through holding white childhood "pure" and nonwhite childhood "suspect," childhood is positioned as an uneven terrain, dependent less on age than on race, class, and global location. "Innocence," including the presumed sexual innocence of asexuality, becomes routinely attributable more to white bodies and white children than to brown and black bodies and children. Asexuality-as-ideal, drawing on Hawkins Owen, is thus caught up in this embrace of rendering whiteness innocent.[19] At the same time, protectionist discourses of people of color as "childish" have been mobilized historically to justify enslavement, oppression, and white supremacy.[20] Notions of preserving "innocence" have also been mobilized to justify the unethical treatment of people with disabilities, such as in the case of Ashley X, a young white girl with disabilities who received hormone treatment, a mastectomy, and a hysterectomy, intended to align her body with her purported "cognitive age."[21] Thinking about asexuality as an ideal that is imposed unevenly in conjunction with discourses of racial innocence provides some insight on childhood as a complex site for navigating injustice.[22]

There have been many creative responses to the desexualization of childhood and children. Freudian psychoanalysis, relying on white notions of futurity and ableist ideas of sexuality, presents the white child as a robustly sexual being. Freud's child is a site of sexual desire from early infancy, and perhaps even prior to this, in utero.[23] As I explored in the introduction, Freud held eros to be at the base of all action in the world, understanding eros as directly grounded in libido and the sexual drive.[24] The infant is formulated by Freud as a tangle of sexual nerves, "polymorphously perverse," and experiencing its whole body as a site of sexual satisfaction.[25] It is only through socialization that the child forms "mental dams" such as disgust, shame, and morality that prevent it from pursuing certain forms of sexual pleasure.[26] Bodily and interbodily acts such as suckling, pooing, being bathed, changed, burped, and held are all understood, psychoanalytically, as being not only sites of pleasure for the infant, but sites of sexual pleasure that then lay the foundation for the process of development and maturation, sexual differentiation into two genders, and entry into the world of subjects.[27] Also, as Freud's family sagas suggest, the child is necessarily sexually entangled with others, implicated in sexual alignments with mothers and fathers. In this psychoanalytic sense, then, the child desexualized is a child torn away from the basic coordinates of self-making, subjectivity formation, and relationality.

Understood in another way, the Freudian child is not only a sexual receiver, that is, a site of sexual enjoyment and experience, but also a sexual provider, providing sexual gratification to the mother and to others from conception onward. Experiences of pregnancy, of birth, and of breastfeeding have all been described at times as sexually erotic, as causing orgasm, pleasure, pain.[28] In this sense, the child is sexual not only in that, psychoanalytically understood, it is a receptor of sexual pleasure, but also as a being that from its inception stimulates sexual pleasure in others. To desexualize a child in this reading is to also cut adults off from the innate corporeal sexual pleasures that nurturing children provides while generating guilt and shame for feeling sexual sensations.

Building on psychoanalysis, queer theory strives also to claim the child's innate right to sexual desire and pleasure, and all that this encompasses. De-desexualizing children insists on challenging what Eve Sedgwick usefully marked as the "systematic separation of children from queer adults" in a society that "wants its children to know nothing; wants its queer children to conform . . . or die."[29] In other words, queer theory is invested in encouraging children to know and claim their queerness through being exposed to sexual knowledge and cultures. This project of de-desexualizing childhood stretches in several directions, but includes arguments for nuanced sex education (as opposed to abstinence-based sex education); more intricate thinking around intergenerational sexual practices and acts; and an approach to children's bodies that does not involve slapping the hand of the masturbating child but rather facilitates sexual self-knowledge, awareness, and possibility for sexual pleasure. More recently, work on temporality from transgender, crip, and critical race perspectives has raised questions as to who exactly queer theory has in mind when "the child" is invoked. Muñoz, for example, has drawn attention to the ways the child of queer theory is a white child, enveloped in discourses of innocence, purity, and entitlement.[30] Ellen Samuels, on the other hand, points out that "impassioned discussions of queer temporalities and queer futurity in the past several years have proceeded as if people with disabilities, queer or otherwise, do not exist."[31] These critiques and others point to the ways in which whiteness and ability are established as unspoken principles from which queer theoretical engagements with childhood have stemmed.

Another unspoken principle from which queer theory has unfolded is the presumed inherentness of sexual desire. Steven Angelides in "Feminism, Child Sexual Abuse, and the Erasure of Child Sexuality" (2004), for instance, talks of desexualization specifically in terms of asexuality, suggesting the degree to which there is a semantic slippage between the two.[32] Looking in particular at feminist literature on sexual assault and children, Angelides argues against the "rigorous attempts to conceal, repress, or ignore the reality and dynamics of child sexuality" as a form of violence to children.[33] Slipping in and out of the language of "desexualization" and "asexuality," Angelides undertakes the important rhetorical moves of arguing against the categorical separation of "childhood" and "adulthood." Yet childhood "asexuality" is collapsed by Angelides with "sexual innocence," described as "asexual innocence," and spoken of in terms of "childhood innocence"—such as in the depiction of the "sexual adult and the asexual child."[34] In other words, asexuality is consistently invoked as a space of "innocence." This account implicitly relies on notions of childhood that are invested in the neutrality and presumed innocence of whiteness as well as developmental narratives about the importance of sexual desire to subject formation. This joining of asexuality with innocence ascribes it a status different from everything else, the sexual somehow existing as its own type, quality, or specialness of experience within the "fallacy of misplaced scale."[35]

Asexuality is rendered throughout Angelides's piece as both impossible and devoid of content, as well as unjust and suffocating for children. This clean slide between asexuality and desexualization is such that asexuality cannot and is not imagined as a desirable, or even as a possible state among children, let alone adults. The message that surfaces is that sexual desires and experiences are a positive, recuperating, queer force, whereas asexuality is a conservative, potentially violent dictum that prevents children from being whole. At the same time, contexts of growing into asexuality, whether through trauma, incest, sexual violence, or a disinterest in sex, are left beyond the frame. Relying on an abstract imaging of the child as white, cisgender, able-bodied, and sexual, childhood is invoked more as a theoretical terrain than as a variegated process lived through on uneven terms. As part of this queer temporality, the sexual surfaces as the only possible mode of queer relating and desiring, leaving behind possibilities for nonsexual and asexual queerness. Upon reading the piece, I was left to wonder: Where are the asexuals of queer theory?—those prudish queers who practice queerness through asexuality and nonsexuality, who are either born not wanting or who mature, gloriously, into not wanting?

An absence of affirmative asexual renderings within queer theory, as I am fleshing out with the figure of the child, is suggestive of a continued attachment to some sexual acts and desires being rendered queer, transgressive, political, and others being rendered not queer, not transgressive, not political. Leo Bersani, Yasmin Nair, Annamarie Jagose, and others have critiqued the continued insistence on making certain sexual acts queerly political: that is, "the longing to maintain some relation between sexual practice and social change."[36] So, for instance, Bersani argued against this equating of particular acts with radicality by assessing that "to want sex with another man is not exactly a credential for political radicalism" because it can be accompanied with bourgeouisiness, racism, or gentrification.[37] Similarly, Nair writes that "your sex is not radical. Your politics can and should be. Consider the difference, and act upon it."[38] Sex and politics are conjoined, but the "ways in which having sex politicizes are highly problematic," or at least ambiguous.[39] Also, as Jagose makes clear with her inventive exploration of the fake orgasm, some sex acts, practices, or identities are accorded queer prestige and cache, while others simply are not, because of the troubling implications they might carry for queerness or politics.[40]

Scavenging from Jagose, we could say that nonsexualities, asexualities, and especially the queer figure of the asexual child have "the potential to estrange us productively from our more familiar knowledges about the relations between erotic practice and the desire for social transformation."[41] This is not to suggest that asexuality can trouble queer theory, but to reflect, as I have been doing, on the manner in which asexuality is painted as irrelevant. Indeed, nonsexuality, and all the practices, modes, and terms that might fall under this umbrella—asexuality, lesbian bed death, political celibacy/asexuality, celibacy, virginity, abstinence—appear to be misbehaving (perverse?) erotic objects, concepts, identities when it comes to queer theory. They serve as deposit sites for backwardness, antisociality, conservativism, and prudery and are held suspect for anti-queer sentiment.

I am suggesting that queer theoretical commitments to the child as definitively and universally sexual (that is, desiring sex and focused on attaining sexual pleasure) come to constitute their own particular imposition on children, the figure of the child, and on how we understand ourselves as adults. Because "the child and its sexuality are . . . already known and knowable . . . queer theory . . . is the advocate of a true knowledge of the child and sexuality" that falls into the same traps it identifies in the paradigm of childhood desexualization.[42] This unquestioned assumption of children's sexuality is a sexual presumption that continues to take broad strokes in regard to the diverse and asymmetrical experiences of subjects who fall within the category of "childhood." It is invested in a particular developmental narrative that draws on the temporal orders established through a white colonialism interested in smoothing out development toward the reproduction of fit bodies in heterosexual contexts. In salvaging childhood from asexuality, the ways in which children's experiences of desire, racialization, class, ability, trauma, and gender—not to mention diverse cultural contexts—come to constitute children in varying relations to sex and to sexuality are lost.

Further, both sides of the desexualization debate—both the "sexual purity" side as much as the "sexual agency" side of debating children's rights either *to* sexuality or *from* sexuality, respectively—are fundamentally tied to a model of development that sees sexual desire as the natural, primal, primary, and preferred outcome. Within the "sexual purity" model, which saves children from sexuality through notions of white innocence, sexual development is deferred, its arrival precipitated by adulthood. Within arguments against desexualization, including queer and psychoanalytic ones, sexual arrival is part and parcel of childhood and does not predate adulthood, yet whiteness is still assumed as an unexamined standpoint from which childhood is theorized. Both models of approaching children's sexualities are joined in an expectation that development and maturation rests upon becoming sexually desiring beings and draws on a logic of white temporality. Both sides of the polarized childhood debate thus rest on a sexual presumption, a framing that renders asexuality ultimately unthinkable as a positive site of identity. In short, queer theory's claim to children's right to be sexual is primarily a moral claim; that is, it is a wish that it were so because of sex's key standing within queer theory itself.

## QUEER CHILDHOOD EROTICS BEYOND SEX

What would take place if queers did not wish for children to be sexual? How would adult viewings of children alter if we did not approach them with a sexual presumption? Notably, this is not to be understood as supporting a desexualization of children, but rather as an opportunity for fleshy and bodily relatings to not be distilled to the sexual, leaving no imaginable space for asexual children. In other words, if queer children are "straightened" through censorship of queer knowledge, banning of queer community, pathologization, and brutality, who is to say that asexual children are not also being coerced into sexual development, under the presumption that sexual desire and sex are inevitable and necessary for "development"?

In this portion of the chapter, I will explore Maggie Nelson's "auto-theoretical" text *The Argonauts* (2015), which provides provocative resolutions for making sense of intergenerational erotics.[43] I see *The Argonauts* as a tract on intergenerational erotics that provides a dishevelment of desexualized white childhood and white motherhood. The questions that drive this consideration are as follows: What would an asexual development narrative look like? How can we make asexual development tangible without desexualizing childhood?

*The Argonauts,* Maggie Nelson's ninth book, is a creative nonfiction memoir—dubbed "auto-theory"—that navigates questions of queer feminist lived embodiment across experience-informed theorizations of sex, identity, community, desire, and motherhood.[44] I am interested, particularly, in how Nelson frames the intergenerational erotics of mothering in a way that may speak to a developmental narrative that does not ostracize asexuality in pursuit of an assumed, ever-present, and ever-transgressive sexuality. *The Argonauts* (2015) is, in turn, a work that makes and unmakes identities and the reliance on conceptualizations of transgression and normativity that underwrite them. The title, referential of Roland Barthes and of Sedgwick's formulation of "queer," hints at this play between the making and unmaking of self, or love, or queerness, or writing for that matter, since the *Argo* "is a boat whose parts are renewed over time, even as its name remains the same."[45]

Nelson creates slivers of possibilities for asexual development, for asexual childhood, and for a desuturing of sex and sexuality from queerness. While it is true that the same might be said of many queer texts if read against their own grain for "asexual resonances," I turn to Nelson's text because it thinks queerness through childhood and motherhood and is in direct conversation with Catherine Opie, whose work I examine in the final section.[46] Nelson's text curates its very own compendium of intergenerational love, including literary critic Jane Gallop's photographs with her son by husband Dick Blau; Susan Fraiman's sodomitical motherhood; Freud's case study of the "Wolf Man," who witnessed his parents-at-sex doggy style; and A. L. Steiner's installation *Puppies and Babies* (2012).[47]

The space of "mother" is here not a gender-determined one, since "one of the gifts of genderqueer family making—and animal loving—is the revelation of caretaking as detachable from—and attachable to—any gender, any sentient being."[48] At the same time, Nelson immerses us in the fleshy, titular, and messy experience of various forms of mothering, including but not limited to the deep pain of the birthing mother, the mother at play with her stepson, the desiring "sodomitical mother,"[49] the "good enough mother" (from Donald Winnicott),[50] and the mother-as-methodology for writing. As with gender, Nelson renders mothering to be many things simultaneously.

In writing childhood, Nelson is always writing of the particularities of the children around her—mostly those of her stepson and her newborn, Iggy. Around the body of Iggy in particular, she articulates an erotics, "but even an erotics feels too heavy. I don't want an eros, or hermeneutics, of my baby. Neither is dirty, neither is mirthful, enough."[51] Erotics is clearly the word I am caught on, speaking as it does to my hopes of imagining forms of relating and desiring that are amenable to asexuality. Nelson's intergenerational erotics/non-erotics of parent and child are suggestive of an intimacy that is neither distinctly sexual nor asexual: "It is romantic, erotic, and consuming—but without tentacles. I have my baby, and my baby has me. It is a buoyant eros, an eros without teleology."[52] Nelson further writes:

> I was so in awe of Iggy's fantastic little body that it took a few weeks for me to feel that I had the right to touch him all over. . . . [T]he culture's worrying over pedophilia in all the wrong places at times made me feel unable to approach his genitals or anus with wonder and glee, until one day I realized, he's my baby, I can—indeed I must!—handle him freely and ably. My baby! My little butt! Now I delight in his little butt. . . . Luckily, Iggy couldn't care less.[53]

Leading me back to the scene of my own family's butt exposure, I hear Nelson speaking to a way of seeing the child's body that is driven by wants and desires, needs, the musts of touching, of handling, of loving that is not precisely sexual, that is joyous in its indefatigable fleshy contact. Nelson's ode to Iggy's little butt is met, on the other hand, with an indifference from Iggy, who "couldn't care less" in his very own little asexually indifferent mode, and yet so clearly requires that touch and fleshy contact, for even if "bodies do not remember being held well—what they remember is the traumatic experience of not being held well enough."[54]

It is in part Nelson's tendency to write and then to unwrite her writing, her movement toward doubt, that makes it possible for asexual developmental possibilities to slip in. Of her writing process, Nelson indicates that it "is riddled with . . . tics of uncertainty. I have no excuse or solution, save to allow myself the tremblings, then go back in later and slash them out. In this way I edit myself into a boldness that is neither native nor foreign to me."[55] Yet because the "tics of uncertainty" are not edited out in full, asexuality and nonsexualities can find their way onto the page.

While there are few specific examples that I can pull of asexual development in Nelson's writing, since I really do not think that asexuality is on her political horizon in *The Argonauts* (2015), there is something about her writing and unwriting, as about her political commitments to a capacious queerness that creates an atmosphere hospitable to asexuality. Politically, Nelson is strongly invested, as I mentioned, in a doing and undoing of identity that requires a questioning of the bounds and forms of transgression and normativity and its uses: "No one set of practices or relations has the monopoly on the so-called radical, or the so-called normative."[56]

The most asexually resonant moment in Nelson's text is the claiming of motherly fatigue as a nonsexual erotics that has as much claim to queerness as any sexually overinvested practice might. "Now," she writes, "I think we have a right to our kink and our fatigue, both."[57] The "now" of this statement, the claiming of fatigue as a legitimate nonsexual space that pushes sex to the side, is for me reminiscent of Valerie Solanas's statement (from the first chapter) that SCUM women (like Solanas herself) emerge and develop into asexuality rather than away from it. Solanas wrote: "Funky, dirty, low-down SCUM gets around . . . [T]hey've seen the whole show—every bit of it. . . . [Y]ou've got to go through a lot of sex to get to anti-sex, and SCUM's been through it all, and they're now ready for a new show."[58] As Breanne Fahs writes, "the basic assumption behind Solanas's glorified asexuality is this: one must experience a lot of sex before arriving at anti-sex. One should not simply become asexual as a means to preserve innocence, virginity, or purity; rather, asexuality is a consequence of sexuality, the logical conclusion to a lifetime of 'Suck and Fuck.'"[59] While, as I mentioned in the first chapter on the feminist celibacy/asexuality of the women's movement, the asexuality Solanas articulates, and the asexuality that Fahs sees in Solanas, are distinct from contemporary asexual identity and community, there is a cousined relationship between these nonsexualities insofar as they are both met with suspicion within compulsory sexuality, or a context that seeks to erase or devalue them.[60]

Leaving this question presently aside, what I want to tease out is the way in which Solanas and Nelson both present possibilities for an asexual development—a growing into asexuality as opposed to a growing up and out of or beyond asexuality. If, as Milks argues, "asexuality is constructed as an immature, underdeveloped, and incomplete form of pre-sexuality suffering from stunted growth," then Nelson's sexual fatigue and Solanas's sexual refusal both suggest the reverse.[61] Speaking to narratives that desexualize childhood and present asexuality as a childish space we should all grow out of, Nelson and Solanas both reverse this developmental model by suggesting that asexuality and other nonsexualities could be something that we grow into.

*Growing into* rather than *out of* asexuality upsets the dominant models of childhood development that I have been examining through this chapter. Rather than "arrested" or "stunted," which are so strongly permeated with a temporality of development rooted in ableism, colonialism, whiteness, and homophobia, growing into asexuality leaves space to think about how trauma, desire, and life itself interrupt processes of heteronormative life progression. Growing into is a rather empowering term in the sense that it neither negates the past nor lets the past predetermine the present; rather, growing into suggests a process of growth and of becoming. To grow into asexuality is to find a point of concord between oneself, one's body, and the erotic dynamics one is enmeshed in. Further, this framing refuses to equate asexuality with loss or inadequacy and to draw on ableist and racist language of being temporally frozen in time, delayed in development. It suggests that asexuality could be a desirable site to grow into. It also suggests that asexuality could arise as a site of rest after years of "suck and fuck" (as for Solanas) or as a form of queer fatigue (as for Nelson). In such a way, for Nelson, sex-positive sodomitical mother that she is, "exchanging horniness for exhaustion grows in allure."[62] Asexuality as exhaustion or fatigue again speaks to those darker affective structures that I laid out in the previous chapter and their robust refusal of homo-/heteronormativity. A fatigued asexuality speaks differently to me than ideals of white virtuous motherhood that inscribe asexuality as an ideal because it speaks to the failings of the maternal body and to the sapping of energies that reproduction requires. Even more so, a fatigued asexuality, following Nelson, could also be a fatigue toward the sex-positive inclinations of queer politics—that is, a queer fatigue.

Further, having "a right to our . . . fatigue" and having "seen the whole show . . . the fucking scene, the sucking scene, the dyke scene" also suggest a threat to a queer developmental model that sees sexuality as ever-present throughout the life cycle, and as central to maintaining the bonds of queer community.[63] Nelson explores the fulcrum that holds sexuality as the site of transgression and cause of celebration within queerness: "What sense does it make to align 'queer' with 'sexual deviance,' when the ostensibly straight world is having no trouble keeping pace? . . . If queerness is about disturbing normative sexual assumptions and practices, isn't one of these that sex is the be-all and end-all?"[64] It is in this questioning of sex and that possibility of holding on to sexual fatigue or disinterest that a queer space hospitable to asexuality and all other forms of nonsexuality takes form. The child and the mother emerge in a relationship that is both sexual and asexual and amenable to queer asexual erotics that step out of white temporal orders of development and delay.

## THE TIME SPELLS OF QUEER AND TRAUMATIC INTERGENERATIONAL EROTICS

In this final section, I develop another model for thinking about intergenerational erotics as a site permeated with asexuality by exploring Catherine Opie's *Self-Portrait/Nursing* (2004) and *Self-Portrait/Cutting* (1993) and Vivek Shraya's photo essay *Trisha* (2016) (see figure 3.1).[65] I want to suggest that both artists queer notions of child-adult sexunormative temporality by elaborating erotic forms that provide reflection on the intimacies of parenting and being parented. Specifically, while Nelson and Solanas imply that asexuality is something that one grows into rather than out of, Opie's and Shraya's work lingers in the "time spells" that parenting and being parented in proximity to trauma provides, an intergenerational erotics neither self-evidently sexual nor asexual.

Motherhood, the most perverse of all intimacies, entangled as it is with a blurring of bodily edges and boundaries, and resting on an unequal, intense intergenerational intimacy, is nonetheless held ideologically as a site of pure "asexual" love.[66] In this sense, motherhood and childhood, both, are enshrined culturally in ideals of asexuality, ideals that comprehend asexuality as purity, innocence, devotion. Yet innocent love is here rendered white, while racialized motherhood is, as Roberts argues in regard to black motherhood, rendered "inherently unfit and even affirmatively harmful to their children"—a love that is not "pure."[67] An asexual ideal of motherhood is entangled in this way in "the privileging of bourgeois, white, patriarchal, and heteronormative ideals and aspirations—such as sexual purity, domesticity, and Puritan morality."[68] White motherhood can retain its claim to both purity and to an asexual ideal, and claim itself as "worthy" of protection, for the reason that racialized womanhood and motherhood are rendered suspect or sullied by sexuality.[69]

Additionally, Hawkins Owen argues that "asexuality-as-ideal" is utilized by whiteness. She writes that through a "misinterpretation of asexuality as the honorable achievement or performance of sexual restraint; the white practitioner is considered pure and deserving of reverence, while the black asexual figure [i.e., the figure of the mammy] is considered less threatening than her hypersexual counterpart [i.e., the figure of the jezebel]."[70] Following philosopher Charles W. Mills, Hawkins Owen identifies whiteness as a set of power relations—that is, not so much an attribute of the body as of a history of sedimented exchanges between bodies.[71] Whiteness, as a racist project, continues to hold asexuality, including a masculine asexuality, as either "revered" (such as in the case of clerical celibacy, where men exert control over their bodies toward attaining bodily purity) or "grievable" (such as in the sense of the loss of white virile masculinity).[72] Ideals of white asexual motherhood and white asexual childhood, then, operate under the sign of a sexual presumption, an expectation that both mothers and children will develop or return to a sexual space, suspended for the present due to ideas of white purity and greater good. Asexuality appears as a desire of racial purity, a desire for white mastery, and an accomplishment attributable to whiteness. In this sense, white motherhood is configured as a morally upright position that is to be emulated but never achieved by racialized mothers.

Representations of white children in the mainstream commonly model themselves on ideas of the desexualized child, rehearsing expectations as to proper intergenerational engagement between adults and children and around appropriate touch between parenting adults and parented children. Naked children are in turn perceived as sexualized, their innocence "corrupted." Catherine Opie's work challenges this santitized erotics of parenting through reflecting more deeply on the ambivalent spaces between love, sexual love, and erotic attachment.

Opie's now renowned work in *Self-Portrait/Nursing* (2004) and *Self-Portrait/Cutting* (1993) offers a hypnotic reflection on desire, erotics, parenting, and the limits of whiteness.[73] Opie's art occupies a rare position in art history as it is both renowned or even mainstreamed as an exemplar of "queer" (or "lesbian") art as well as inherently sub- and countercultural, legible to queer viewers and speaking back against homophobia, sex negativity, and the suppression of queer and BDSM cultures. Taken ten years apart, *Self-Portrait/ Cutting* and *Self-Portrait/Nursing* enact desires for queer family in the face of trauma and a homophobic society that refused to warrant nonheterosexual family structures. *Cutting* (1993) features a photograph of Opie's back freshly dripping blood from a recently etched image of two stick figure women holding hands under a partially cloud-obscured sun and next to a house. Opie's bleeding back is set against an almost opulent dark-green wallpaper with a frieze of knotted fabric and florals.[74] In *Nursing* (2004), Opie's dreams are perhaps met as she is handling a past-breastfeeding-age child with one of her etchings ("Pervert") light but visible on her chest.[75] Again set against an opulent backdrop, this time one of ruby-red flowing sheets with golden florals, Opie looks down serenely at her breastfeeding child while securely holding him in place with both her hands placed under his body. The scene here is reminiscent of Madonna and Child imagery present in Catholic symbolism from the fifth century onward, in which a devout mother looks upon the child in her arms in an act of intimacy. Read from a current day standpoint through a liberal lens in the chronological sequence of their creation, the two photographs might suggest dreams achieved over a homonormative passing of time or, through a conservative lens, they might suggest the successful "perverting" of culture and queer contamination of parenting. Yet, when examined in reverse, *Nursing* and *Cutting* speak to the ongoing nature of past dreams and traumas, and the unclear distinction between sexual and asexual forms of erotics.

Nude white children, especially when in the embraces of nude adults, are often prone to being read through a "pedophilic gaze" in a context that, on the one hand, is attached to the mythologies of compulsory sexuality within the context of "healthy" and able-bodied adulthood and on the other hand holds asexuality as an ideal of whiteness.[76] Opie's *Nursing* tells a story of white children's development that is disturbing to many audiences as it constitutes an unnerving confrontation of asexual ideals of pure white childhood. Violating an unspoken code around how white children should be cared for and breastfed, the developmental narrative that is conveyed is one that aligns with queer theory's wish for childhood to be sexual. Yet studying this image, I am not altogether sure whether it is that the "sexual" is a property of the photographs and not an effect of their circulation in a context of compulsory sexuality that, while denying sexuality to children through desexualization, nonetheless holds it as a central determinant of identity later in life. *Nursing*, in distinction to its takeup and circulation, instead holds open the possibility for an intergenerational erotics that is not exactly sexual, if not exactly asexual either.

Maggie Nelson writes that Opie's *Self Portrait/Nursing* and in particular "the ghosted [pervert] scar offers a rebus of sodomitical maternity," connecting maternity/parenthood to queer cultures.[77] Opie's *Nursing* positions queer desires for family as against homonormative time sequencing, infusing perversion and "sodomitical maternity" into the frame. While understood as asserting the sexual space of lesbianism and queer culture through references to BDSM, both photographs direct our attention to the blurriness of what might qualify as "the sexual" in the first place, gesturing toward an erotics that is not encompassable by sexual desire, framing queerness as about an erotic desire for parenting, community, and family, and in a sense challenging rather than reinstating a queer focus on sex and sexual desire.

Undertaking the reverse reading of the parent-child erotic, Vivek Shraya's *Trisha* (2016) explores the complex longings that daughterhood facilitates through expounding her desires for her own mother. Shraya is a Canadian-raised South Asian transfeminine artist who creates across mediums, including through music, film, creative writing in multiple genres, and photography. In the photo essay *Trisha* (2016), Shraya staged nine photographs that link her, across time, space, and context, to photographs of her mother from the 1970s. In turn, each photo couplet includes a photo of her mother and a photo of herself, with a careful composition that rehearses and reframes the clothing, setting, and postures of her mother's photographs. For example, in one photograph, Shraya is in the kitchen cutting a cake; in another talking on the phone while leaning against a wood-paneled wall; and in another, an analog lens filter features her reflected five times over in a red dress resting in a lawn chair (see figure 3.1).

The series explores Shraya's love and longing for her mother as well as the effects this has had on her own femininity. The mother's desires and the daughter's desires brush up and interconnect with one another toward seeking to resolve the knowledge that mothers sacrifice parts of themselves for their children and that children also sacrifice parts of themselves for their mothers. Shraya reflects on the ways in which her mother looked happy and light in the photos in a way she had never known her to be because of the struggles that beat down immigrant mothers, namely overwork, overmothering, racism, displacement, and spirit injury. Shraya writes, "I remember finding these photos of you three years ago and being astonished, even hurt, by your joyfulness, your playfulness. I wish I had known this side of you, before Canada, mar-

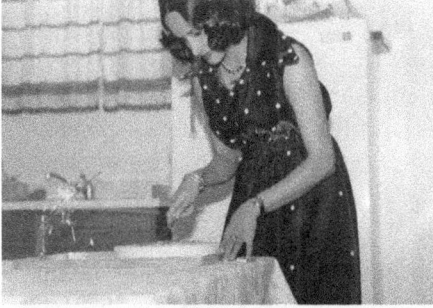

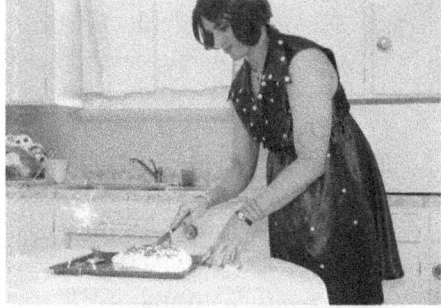

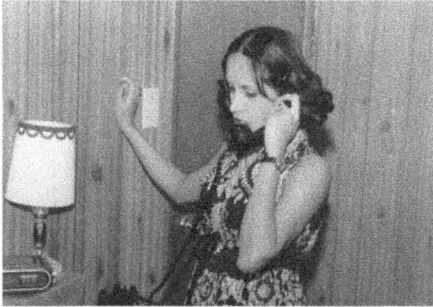

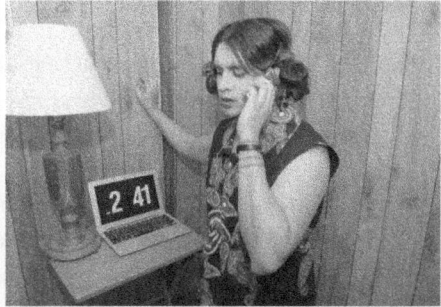

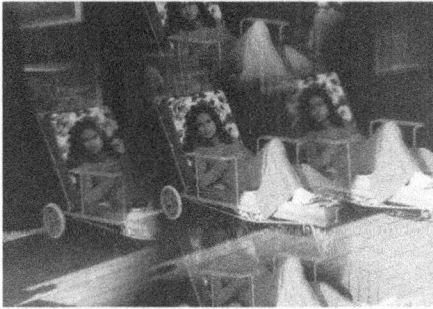

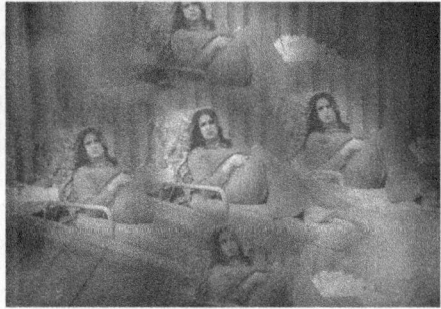

**FIGURE 3.1.** Vivek Shraya, *Trisha*, 2016. Copyright and courtesy of the artist. https://vivekshraya.com/visual/trisha/.

riage and motherhood stripped it from you, and us."[78] If Opie's work reflects on queer perverse desires for parenting and the ambiguously a/sexual erotics of intergenerational love, Shraya's *Trisha* is a tribute to the longings of being a child desiring a certain erotics that our parents sometimes cannot provide. Desiring a certain mother that has been lost or at least altered through the hardships of immigrant mothering in racist contexts, Shraya expresses a yearning for being with her mother in ways that might not be feasible. She in return resolves these desires through recreating her mother's photographs, giving herself and her mother the joyous erotics that life circumstance might have curtailed.

Both artists theorize intergenerational erotics through a "time spells" temporality whereby the bodies featured in the art travel between past and present, exploring the persistence of desires past. Opie's work suggests the persistent effects of wounding and scarring, blurring the lines of pain and healing. Through a similar framing of the two photographs, Opie implies a continuity between the queerness of wounding and the queerness of parenting, and the viewer time travels between one moment and the next. The temporal frame in Shraya's series likewise constitutes a persistence of the past in the present moment; the desires and longings of Shraya's mother are with her, transmitted intergenerationally. Whereas, as Kathryn Bond Stockton argued in *The Queer Child, or Growing Sideways in the Twentieth Century* (2009), development is "relentlessly figured as vertical movement upward (hence, 'growing up') toward full stature, marriage, work, reproduction, and the loss of childishness," both artists challenge this temporal order through experimenting with time spells.[79] Time spells are in this sense an artist's invitation to viewers to travel with them, creating alternate temporal orders than those encountered under the staightening effects of capitalism, heteronormativity, and colonialism.

Time spells are also the stuff of trauma and both artists' work reflects on the time spell effects of trauma as homophobia, transphobia, racism, and displacement create conditions of parenting and being parented that make time circular, redundant, and the past present. Clementine Morrigan, discussing trauma and childhood abuse, points out the unique temporal structure of "trauma time" as nonlinear time, not a procession from past to present toward the future, but rather as involving breaks in remembering and a flooding of memories that feel present rather than past.[80] In both Opie's and Shraya's art, there is evidence of these time spells, as postures and settings are revisited and sequenced. These erotic time spells are neither sexual nor asexual; rather, they occupy a distinct muddied terrain that is about desires, longings, and pain.

Yet despite the similar ways in which Opie and Shraya put forward an intergenerational erotics that reflects on trauma and is not bound to sexuality, each series does so by way of making a different set of postulations around racialization. In Opie, as I explored, the "innocence" afforded to white childhood is challenged, yet also drawn on as a resource in upholding the tender moment evident in *Nursing*, referential as it is of a virginal-style imagery of a revered motherhood. In Shraya's work, intergenerational erotics are not voiced through a play of the false conflation of whiteness with innocence but through a framework of brown diasporic longing. José Esteban Muñoz described the ways in which brownness, in relation to but not limited to Latinx identity, is constituted as a set of affects distinct from those of hegemonic whiteness— that is, as "feeling brown."[81] White affective structures are constituted through manners of temporal distribution and rhythms of behavior: the role of acting white that is so formative to practices of whiteness as dominance. In this sense, it could be argued that Opie's *Nursing* subtly challenges white modes of conduct through breastfeeding past appropriate age, imbibing "innocent" white motherhood with "sodomitical" intentions, all while retaining some form of reference to a virginal-type form of motherhood and the stable family unit based on intergenerational erotics, love, and commitment. Shraya's series, on the other hand, challenges the temporality of racialized immigration whereby the parents are assumed to hang on to the traditions and dress of one's culture while the children are assumed to adopt and want to adopt the dress codes and affects of the hegemonic white culture. Instead, Shraya's *Trisha* visits and remakes "feeling brown," challenging the temporal framing of immigration as a path to assimilating to white patterns, dress codes, and affects. Instead of the temporal story of immigrant assimilation, Shraya's work engages in a time spells temporality, subverting this order of supposed growth into white culture and away from one's parents' cultural affects and desires.

Further, rather than the "before and after" frameworks of visual gender transition stories—which often espouse a form of celebration for their subjects as to the bodily changes that have taken place—Shraya's series enacts a different temporal mode of transition. Sheila Cavanagh, drawing on psychoanalyst Bracha Ettinger, calls this the "Other sexual difference" or woman-to-woman difference in which "Shraya's narration of her transition is less about becoming feminine (in fact, she says she was never masculine, but soft)" and more about thinking about herself as feminine in similarity and difference to her mother.[82] Rather than a before and after of the body, the transition story is one of the ongoingness of the past in the present through "time spells," revisiting the self through one's mother, a mother one does not recognize. *Trisha*, the name Shraya's mom would have given to a child assigned female at birth, is the name of the series—the name less so of Shraya herself than of the desires and longings that feed intergenerational erotics and the impossibility of parents and children, both, to live up to each others' expectations in situations of duress. Transitioning in this series is thus not about telling a story of bodily progress, assimilation, or even relationship progress but about drawing attention to the sticky persistence of desires and how they shape intergenerational erotics within conditions of trauma.

Queer theorist Elizabeth Freeman outlines "erotohistoriography" as "a politics of unpredictable, deeply embodied pleasures that counters the logic of development," in particular in relation to the narrative of past, present, and future.[83] This seems to me an apt way to conceptualize both Opie's and Shraya's work, which touches on the ways that—both representationally and through parenting—"a woman is a partner in an erotic relationship with a child."[84] As I have explored in the introduction to this book, I am holding on to erotics as a term that offers possibilities distinct from sexuality.[85] Erotics speak to forms of relating that are in excess of sexuality in the sense that sexuality's possibilities are determined by its harnessing into biopolitical and neoliberal organizations of space, time, and bodies. Erotics are suggestive for me of an alternate mode through which to imagine bodily proximity, and the pleasure or desire flows that might or might not be associated with them. Erotohistoriography, in this sense, becomes about tracing the asexual intimacies and forms of representation that trouble sexually presumptive schemes of development.

To say that Opie's and Shraya's work is "erotic" but perhaps not sexual is thus a way to broaden the terms on which parenting is understood. As a form of intergenerational erotics, parenting is neither sexual nor asexual, but rather entangled in the complexity of affective registers common to any form of relating. To say that Opie's work in particular is erotic is to challenge both conservative claims that it "sexualizes" childhood or motherhood as well as queer celebrations of childhood sexuality. Hence, childhood and intergenerational erotics make feasible desires that are not easily distilled to a sexual presumption. Within *Nursing* and *Cutting* as well as *Trisha*, the time frames of motherhood/parenting, trauma, and desire are blurred through "time spells," creating an ambiguity around which desires are "sexual" and which are not. Asexual erotics surface instead as a deep desire for presence with those we are erotically entangled with. If Nelson and Solanas postulate a "growing into" asexuality through fatigue and refusal, Shraya's and Opie's work experiments with the asexual erotics that linger around parenting and being parented as a web of desires that informs the intimate, yet not straightforwardly sexual work that goes into mothering and being mothered.

## "WHAT IS OUR LOVING TO CONSIST OF?"[86]

Asexuality is commonly understood in queer readings of the child as doing damage to children, both figurative and real. In the spirit of admitting "that we cannot and must not try to predict in advance what psychological, emotional, and political stories will arise from childhood sexual engagement," I have been arguing that queer readings of childhood must foster an attunement to the possibility of asexual development as a queer model of growth.[87] Queer arguments for children *as sexual* constitute just one example of how asexual and nonsexual identities and developments are actively elided, discounted, and impossibilized in queer articulations. This unchecked reliance on a sexual presumption as a founding, uninterrogated moment of development and queer theory overstates the universality, proclivity, and political prowess of sex and sexuality in intimate queer relating. "What is our loving to consist of?," James Kincaid asks in *Erotic Innocence* (1998)—my niece's and my own—loving each other not through familial obligation but through some other pull?[88] Also, more broadly, "what is our loving to consist of?"—that is, queer theory's loving of sexuality, loving of the child as sexual, and the occasional lack of imagination as to other ways to be queer with each other.[89] How could we articulate intergenerational love, trauma, and erotics, "by positing a *range* of erotic feelings within and toward children [r]ather than assuming that such feelings exist in only two forms—not at all or out of control"?[90] It seems that part of this answer lies with a "complex and dynamic relativity" that is perceptive of the overreliance on sex to do the difficult work of relating for us.[91] Perhaps in thinking relationality, intimacy, and erotics more pliably, queer theory might make space for the type of perversity left unnamed and undesired—for asexualities, nonsexualities.

I will not get around it—my mother might be right; there might be something perverse in my love for my niece, my auntish delight in her silly play or that devilish moment in the morning when she presses her cool hands to my still sleep-warm back. Watching my niece frolic, pants hanging low, I know only that desire—in this case, the intergenerational draw to be kin—is not distillable to the sexual.

# CHAPTER 4

# Erotics of Excess and the
# Aging Spinster

MY MOTHER used to tell me as a child that if I sat at the corner of the table I would become a spinster—an old maid. As I age into my mother's pronouncement, I have been thinking on the economies of aging, the politics of being singled, and what is lost and what is gained by living in a spinsterly way. Most singularly, what erotics have I had the opportunity to unravel due to my spinsterly perversions and delectabilites? In this chapter, I explore the spinsterly and queer erotics of aging as they are entwined with asexuality and desexualization.

The previous chapter explored how childhood is fleshed out by queer scholars as necessarily sexual in an effort to speak back to the constraining forces of desexualization. Desexualization also takes effect on bodies on the opposite end of the age arc, on aging bodies. While childhood is "protected" from sexuality by the forces of desexualization so as to maintain ideals of white purity and innocence, older age is desexualized through a very different discourse. The body altered with time tends to become a site socially despised—rendered ugly in appearance, useless in capitalist schemes of productivity and reproduction, and marked as not worthy and not capable of sexual interest and desire. So, while children and older adults can both be said to be desexualized—that is, structurally and discursively banned from sex—it is through different apparatuses. Childhood is desexualized to protect whiteness, morality—partaking, in short, in a certain will to save white children so as to facilitate their entitled futures. The desexualization of older adults operates on the assumption that aging adults do not have a future, are not worth preserving, are "disposable" and not entitled to pleasure, desire, or sexiness.[1] In the words of Stephen Katz, there is a "[broad] cultural background of contradictory images that marginalize, denigrate, and desexualize older people" even while older adults are enjoined to "resist their own aging through active and independent lifestyles."[2] Yet ideologies of whiteness as a form of sexual superiority continue to inform the desexualization of aging adulthood. Whereas children are desexualized to preserve their "innocence," aging adults discursively stand as symbols of a lifetime of sexual accomplishment who can then depart and retire from the realm of sexual desire whether or not they actually wish to do so.

In this chapter, I will think about the structural and discursive banning of aging adults' sexualities while also maintaining that spinsterly asexuality can provide an erotics that are caught up in both loneliness and joy, an excess of erotics even amidst an absence of sex. I will argue, in particular, that ageism is a politics of disposability, a will to make disappear those deemed discardable by society. I actually do not think that people believe that older adults are "asexual." What I suggest happens instead is that older adults are willed into a nonsexuality that is structurally reinforced—including architecturally, in the layout of nursing homes and long-term facilities—so as to do away with any claims to life and pleasure and reinforce a narrative arc of life grounded in a white disdain of sexuality, or sex negativity. Older adults, held as abject, leaky, dying, and thus as toxic to the spirit and energy of the population more broadly, are forbidden from enjoying their bodies or from forming alliances with other bodies. In this sense, there are conversations to be had between critical disability studies and studies of aging.[3] And as Alison Kafer briefly writes, "anxiety about aging . . . can be seen as a symptom of compulsory able-bodiedness/able-mindedness."[4] In other words, social hatred of both aging bodies and disabled bodies is driven by deep and often unchecked commitments to ideals of youth, health, able-bodiedness, normative beauty, and compulsory sexuality.

Yet, as an asexuality studies scholar, I also want to hold on to the possibility of imagining aging bodies as affirmatively asexual, emphasizing asexual and nonsexual erotics, identities, and experiences as valid and life making. In this sense, I draw on the work of multiple feminists and feminist and queer historians who have sought to think with and for the figure of the spinster. Scholars such as Heather Love, Benjamin Kahan, Peter Coviello, and others have provided us with historical and literary readings of spinsterhood, thickening ideas as to what spinsterhood and being "never married" meant for asymmetrically located women across historical locations.[5] The spinster has also been mobilized as an empowering feminist symbol that speaks to women's independence, talks back to patriarchal contexts, is rife with lesbian erotics, and exists as an effect of being shut out by couple-oriented society. The spinster is a feminist figure of both strength and vulnerability, who, while rendered disposable through a hatred of aging, misogyny, an absence of couple privilege, lack of wealth and cultural resources, and desexualization, nonetheless figures rebelliously throughout history. The spinster is also a white figure of feminist empowerment, as she rests on white bourgeoisie aspirations of singlehood as independence. My chapter adds to this feminist literature by arguing that the spinster is a figure that can be read as affirmatively asexual and excessively erotic. With "the ache of standing outside of things rather than in the midst of them," a spinster is nonetheless open to alternate erotics resonant with asexuality, "build[ing] community wherever she goes" and redefining what it means to be in relation with others.[6] The spinster is a figure as much resonant with loneliness and the desexualization of aging as with inventing ways to survive in a couple-centric society that leaves single women with little space to flourish.

Notably, spinsters are not and have not always been "old," since across historical eras it has been possible to qualify as a spinster from girlhood onward—speaking to the socially and historically inflected categorization of age groups.[7] At the same time, spinsterhood is intimately tied to the idea of the aging body, and to aging femininity in particular, which is perceived as a body running out of reproductive and marital time. In both senses, I can situate myself as a "spinster": as a body on its way to becoming useless from reproductive perspectives and as a queer feminist who homes in on a spinsterly lifestyle and disposition both erotic and lonely. I am curious, thus: What can the figure of the spinster teach us about asexual love, and the joys and loneliness of an aging asexuality?

This chapter proceeds as follows: First, I sketch out what I mean by the concepts of biopolitics, desexualization, and disposability. I find that a conversation around biopolitics is relevant here because it helps us think, at least in an abstract way, of how aging bodies are encouraged to not be sexual, and how this takes effect through various measures that are demeaning to an aging adult's personhood. Dana Luciano has depicted "chronobiopolitics" as "the sexual arrangement of the time of life," and it is useful to think of the desexualization of aging as falling under this arrangement.[8] Using Ranjana Khanna's understanding of disposability, which is grounded in biopolitics, I explore desexualization as a component of biopolitical compulsory sexuality, drawing sparingly on Michel Foucault and Giorgio Agamben.[9] In the second section, I explore how it is that desexualization functions in cohort with other strategies to render older adults, including spinsters, disposable. I will read desexualization through and in concert with architectural arrangements, feeding schedules, thin sociality, and medical touching, to explore how the aging body is produced as disgusting, docile, disposable. Following on this, I will read the spinster recuperatively, drawing on rich feminist attachments to the spinster and similar rebel figures. While it is true that aging adults are desexualized, the spinster is also, I will argue, a figure of excess—erotic excess and in excess of heterosexuality, lesbian relating, and sexual identity categories. The spinster's excess is best understood, in turn, by an asexuality that opens her up onto erotics that are not bound to the desire flows of sex and sexual attracting. Toward this end, my final section will draw on the film *Frances Ha,* directed by Noah Baumbach and written by Baumbach and Greta Gerwig, to flesh out the spinster as an asexual figure of erotic excess.[10] Notably, this analysis of the desexualization of aging, like all the chapters in *Asexual Erotics,* is driven by an asexual reading—that is, this analysis of desexualization, I hold, would not be possible without the activist agitating of the asexual community against claims of dismissal, impossibility, and invisibility and the concomitant academic work on asexuality that likewise strives to argue for the important contributions to be had from thinking sex, sexuality, and relating from asexual perspectives.

## AGING AND DESEXUALIZATION

Compulsory sexuality is biopolitical in the sense that it relies on the insistence that some (the white, healthy, able-bodied, appropriately aging, those with claims to citizenship) should engage in sex, while others (the young, the old, the disabled) should not engage in it. Foucault outlined modern biopower as operating through a "great bipolar technology" that addresses both bodies individually and bodies as populations—that is, biopolitically.[11] Since the intensification of sexuality in the nineteenth century, Foucault holds, and in concord with colonial expansion and slavery, sexuality has functioned to uphold biopower, linking sex to the welfare of the white population both through its "procreative effects" and through the regime of health.[12] This rise of sexuality as a tool of biopower is inherently tied to colonialism and wishes for the health and reproduction of some at the expense and examination of others, and especially of colonized subjects, disabled people, and people understood as deviant or aberrant. In this sense, sexuality has emerged as part of a knowledge project grounded in white supremacy.

Compulsory sexuality, upholding sex and sexuality as central to self-worth, relational formations, and community making, encourages bodies to have sex as part of the project of being healthy, able-bodied, and youthful citizens. Angela Davis writes that compulsory sexuality's operation is racialized such that "while women of color are urged, at every turn, to become permanently infertile, white women enjoying prosperous economic conditions are urged, by the same forces, to reproduce themselves."[13] In this way, the production of desirable populations is biopolitically encouraged even as some groups and bodies are *banned* from sex. Agamben formulates the "ban" as not "simply [being] set outside the law and made indifferent to it but rather abandoned by it, that is, exposed and threatened on the threshold in which life and law, outside and inside, become indistinguishable."[14] Using Agamben's notion of the ban, those who are banned from sex do not lose their sexuality, since they are disposable and their sexuality is beyond sacrifice—that is, you cannot lose something that you are not seen as entitled to in the first place.

Feminist biopolitical theorist Ranjana Khanna, in her discussion of the "contemporaneity of disposable life and death," outlines the manifold meanings of disposability as follows: (1) disposable as in a disposable camera or diaper, which "designates a product created for disposal"; (2) disposable as in disposable income, "something available for use, in excess of notions such as need"; and (3) "the sovereign commandment (over life and death and sexual access)"—that is, the ability to render someone disposable.[15] While "the category of the disposable person is harder to comprehend in terms of these three differentiations," what I take away from Khanna's analysis is that there are "differentiated ways in which life becomes disposable," many of which are caught in capitalist and state-organized machines of production, including the production of citizenship and sexual citizenship.[16] Since, as compulsory sexuality holds, sexual activity and expression are pivotal to one's identity and belonging in modern contexts, desexualization, as a banning of sex to bodies and groups, functions as part of what Foucault terms "letting die."[17]

"Letting die" is the removal of the conditions needed for survival so that bodies and groups of bodies wither, like plants without sun. Desexualization can be considered a mode of letting die in that it entails the spatial, institutional, and discursive repositioning of some bodies, such as the elderly, as not in need of sex because they are, after all, already approaching death, and "old age is taken as synonymous with death—social and actual."[18] Paul Simpson et al. name this "ageist erotophobia," which "defines older people as post-sexual, [and] restricts opportunities for the expression of sexuality and intimacy."[19] At the same time, being able to reach old age is in itself an accomplishment for many whose life is under state erosion since childhood, such as Indigenous people, racialized people, and people with disabilities. Evelyn Reynolds has written that "'aging while black' is an act of survival" because far too often age does not in itself determine when a black person dies due to systemic and institutionalized racism.[20] While stereotypes suggest that "black don't crack" or that black women do not show signs of aging as a means to celebrate black beauty and aging, the reality is that in addition to state-sanctioned violence, the stress of racism increases the chance of life-threatening conditions and premature death.[21] Indeed, Ruth Wilson Gilmore points out pithily that racism is the state-sanctioned production of "group-differentiated vulnerability to premature death," suggesting that it is the design of institutional racism to *not* permit people of color to reach old age in the first place.[22] By extension, discourses around the desexualization of aging, while harmful to all bodies and communities as an imposed framework for discarding the value of maturity and aging, are fundamentally about whiteness. While aging adults are revered in many communities, including in black, Indigenous, and immigrant communities, white colonial society has been invested in diminishing the value of even white aging because of attachments to productivity, reproductivity, and the conflation of youthful beauty with (white) morality. Extending again Ianna Hawkins Owen's work on the racialization of "asexual" discourses, ideas around aging mobilize asexuality as a resource of pristine whiteness, as an accomplishment.[23] In regard to aging, the accomplishment of "asexuality" is the accomplishment not of sexual restraint but of sexual conclusion, of wrapping up one's life project of reproduction and production (and sex) for the nation-state and being able to rest after a job completed. It is within this context of a maturity narrative grounded in whiteness that the desexualization of aging takes effect.

Aging refers to any number of vastly dissimilar experiences structured by variegated social and geographical conditions. For instance, older adults or the elderly span an age difference of over forty years, from sixty-five to upward of one hundred years—age groups shaped by differing eras, politics, values, and life experiences.[24] Older adults are groupable under one category only in the sense that they are discriminated against through a broad "social antipathy towards the elderly" that takes on toxic and life-annihilating forms.[25] This "antipathy," commonly termed ageism, comprises the institutionally sanctioned removal of the right to govern one's body, the loss of social and political status, and the sometimes forced removal from one's home. It is characterized by systemic physical, financial, psychological, and sexual exploitation that includes verbal denigration; ageist hate speech; threats; interception of one's decision-making powers; financial theft and misuse of resources; abuse of financial guardianship; bodily neglect; hitting and pushing; not providing proper nutrition, clothing, and shelter; isolation; lack of necessary medical care and attention; sexual assault; and public humiliation.[26] More than being "vulnerable" to "elder abuse," older adults are produced—discursively, spatially, institutionally—as discardable, disposable. I hold that one way in which aging adults are produced as disposable is through desexualization.

Desexualization functions to dispose of aging adults in at least two broad ways. First, it does so through rendering older adults as sexually undesirable. To be rendered sexually undesirable relies on an intricate and multisensory ableism that picks up on the scents, textures, and appearances of aging and elicits a mode of disgust in those imagined to be youthful. As one sixty-four-year-old lesbian woman who participated in a study that looked at older women's views on sex comments: "I think it's partially because aging is seen as disgusting in this youth culture. And so sex among disgusting beings is even more disgusting."[27] Or as another study that examines college students' attitudes toward aging adults puts forward, the affect of disgust is attached in particular to the sexuality of aging bodies.[28]

Disgust functions as validation for disposability, producing aging bodies as disgusting and banning them from sex.[29] It is thus not so much that the aging body is naturally disgusting, but much more so that it is structured, through the operation of ageism as disgusting so as to keep it in its place—a place of disposability. If the "young" are ill-disposed to the aging, it is because a habitual disgust is cultivated that serves a non-intergenerational project of compulsory sex and sexuality, rendering some bodies sexy and others unfuckable. In turn, the collective use of disgust against aging adults may be considered a biopolitical affect that supports projects of elderly disposal. Since "disgust is an affect that forces us to confront our bodily existence," the displacement of disgust onto the bodies of the elderly through a banning of sex and "sexiness" permits for a deferral of anxieties around aging, bodily change, and senescence.[30]

Notably, the allotment of non-sexiness is especially harmful to women, who are commonly habituated to assessing their value in terms of youth, beauty, and sexiness. The effect of this is the process by which, through a devaluing of their appearance—that is, the loss of their sexiness—a ban against sexual enjoyment is implemented, since "if elderly women can't be beautiful, they obviously can't have sex, either."[31] Also, cisgender women are understood to be disposable in a particular way after they cease to be reproductively useful and capable of procreation.[32] Disability and aging are often tightly linked, as Susan Wendell explores, and while "aging is not always and never *just* being sick or dying . . . it is also these. Aging is also disabling, and especially disabling in societies where inadequate provision is made for the participation of people with nonideal, limited, or suffering bodies."[33] If disgust is a visceral response that points to a desire to maintain bodily boundaries and one's psychic sense of self, then a disgust-based response to aging keeps the segregation of the young and aging in place, facilitating the enactment of compulsory sexuality for the young and young-approximating, and the desexualization of the elderly.[34]

Second, desexualization takes effect through a spatialization of disposability. Sociologist Erving Goffman discussed the "total institution" as "an enclosed, formally administered round of life . . . prison-like . . . whose members [may] have broken no laws."[35] These spaces are tightly scheduled, populated by "a batch of similar others," under ongoing surveillance, where staff and inmates form distinct social groups and the "social mobility between the two strata is grossly restricted."[36] For example, the staff within nursing homes, often overworked and underpaid, prioritize "bed-and-body" work, striving to execute tasks efficiently and abet "the efficient running of the nursing home as a whole."[37] The result of this is the handling of aging adults as a "batch," and the diminishing of opportunities for personalized routines, life habits, and self-expression.[38] Even such aspects as deciding when to eat, whether to shower, when to get out of bed or go outdoors, or what to wear are impossibilized in the "batch living" of a nursing home because individuals are processed as groups rather than as independent agents.[39] Interestingly, while sex could be conceived of as part and parcel of "bed-and-body" work such that it is configured as part of the care of the body, in the current system it is often not.[40] The elderly, when requesting a personalization of the schedule, are instead conceived of by staff as "difficult" or uncooperative, standing in the way of the efficient execution of work tasks in pursuit of "trivialities."[41] The time of the long-term facility or nursing home is in this way "organised around a non-negotiable daily schedule" in which everyday routines are rigidly fixed.[42] The desexualized adult in the long-term facility, banned from basic agency over their body, is rendered passive in a way suitable to the conditions of the total institution. There "are few opportunities for socially dignifying relationships within the nursing home" since elderly adults are plucked out of their home environments and inserted into fabricated communities founded on age segregation—or, as one participant from a recent study commented, they are "warehoused."[43] Care and ethics theorist Joan Tronto argues that "everyone's life . . . is diminished by living in age-segregated circumstances," since it homogenizes the nursing home environment and the community outside the home more broadly.[44]

The space of the long-term facility and nursing home, functions in my analysis to desexualize older adults through the implementation of spatial means that make intimacy and sex nearly inconceivable. The presence of staff, the batch living, the tightly scheduled days, and the constant presence of "similar others" makes for displays of intimacy, including but not limited to sex, difficult and near impossible even for able-bodied elders.[45] Access to sex is prevented through institutional policy, the spatialized absence of privacy, surveillance by similar others and staff, as well as through an absence of personnel who would facilitate access to sex for elders with disabilities or mobility constraints.[46]

For example, a study of the implications on older age sexuality for health care providers depicts an account of two nursing home residents who formed an intimate bond in the form of hand holding and smiling. Because one of the residents was married, "the nurses perceived these interactions as inappropriate and dangerous to Pedro's marriage [and] the decision was made to not place the wheelchairs side-by-side and limit the interaction. They were no longer able to share a touch or smile; shortly after Sue died."[47] In this case, access to intimate interactions was directly intercepted and banned by the staff, demonstrating the extent to which bodily agency is limited and intimacy censored in the desexualization of older adults. Under the guise of "safety," nursing homes are designed to limit privacy with such measures as open-door and no-locked-door requirements and a paucity of single-inhabitant rooms.[48] Also, resident rooms and the space of the nursing home in general compose a space part private, part public, where the very idea of whose "home" it is remains unclear, since staff feel inclined to move through the space freely, compromising the residents' autonomy and privacy.[49] Residents can also be expressly punished for exhibiting whatever is deemed "improper" sexual conduct.[50]

If aging adults are permitted to engage in sex, it is often in consultation with their families, undermining an aging adult's agency over their own body.[51] Family, staff, and managers are thus in the structural position to decide whether one is allowed to engage in sexual activity, effectively dispensing or banning sex at their own whim, as influenced by their own sense of sexual morality and potential ageist attitudes toward older adult sexuality.[52] This position of needing to negotiate sex in a context of widespread desexualization can likewise lead to the practicing of unprotected sex.[53] Queer and transgender people face the additional nullifying of their gender and sexual identities if removed from their homes and placed into long-term care facilities where they may be met with the heterosexual presumption as well as with homophobic and transphobic peers and staff who may refuse to recognize their gender and sexual identities.[54] In this sense, the desexualization of LGBTQ2+ older adults is combined with lethal homophobic and transphobic intent. Indeed, LGBTQ2+ older adults experience entry into the space of the nursing home as particularly alienating, and they experience ongoing nonconscious bias.[55] Through the process of desexualization, older adults are maintained as residents within a facility, without bodily autonomy, and as bodies to be preserved and protected rather than as sites of rich subjectivity entitled to gender and sexual identities.

Widowhood, spinsterhood, and other modes of singlehood are likewise acutely prone to old-age disposability. Unprotected by the structure of couple privilege, single older adults have fewer social structures to prevent their social and sexual diminishment. This affects women disproportionately, since older women are over twice more likely to live alone than older men.[56] Widowhood, for instance, involves the loss not only of a close other but also of the accompanying social networks and sense of belonging.[57] Singlehood in old age also becomes a contributing factor to structural disposability, since one has to resourcefully seek out sex with others in ways that are made difficult due to the rendering of older adults as "unsexy."[58] Widows are also desexualized in specific ways since as "unsexy," they are understood and perhaps understand themselves as lacking the tools necessary to recruit sexual accomplices.[59] As studies show, widowhood is a central deciding factor for whether older adults are sexually active.[60]

Also, adults who are not deemed able-minded may not be legally permitted to offer their own consent, further functioning to ban them from intimate and sexual activities. For instance, residents with dementia in many US states cannot legally partake in sex since they are not viewed as having the "capacity to consent."[61] Sexual activity between a person with dementia or another mental "impairment" may be criminalized, functioning to deprive many adults of autonomy over their bodily lives.[62] Persons with dementia are also held to a higher standard in terms of consent than the general public.[63] A third party or guardian might have decision-making authority over whether an older adult with dementia can partake in sexual activity.[64] In concord with ableism, ageism here functions to ban individuals from sexual intimacy and expression in a context of limited personal freedom and disposability. Significantly, the spaces of aging and disability are overlapping, since the US census suggests that in 2000, 54.7 percent of people over sixty-five had a disability, a number that includes both lifelong and acquired disabilities.[65]

If to be disposable is to have served a purpose and to now be superfluous, the aging body is rendered as having served its reproductive and productive functions, and is thus positioned as of little social value. Unlike the rapture of white childhood futurity, with its unfolding of possible uses, futures, successes, hopes, and aspirations, the aging body promises little capitalist gain even while the narrative of aging deseuxalization continues to be invested in whiteness, white morality, and ideas around the white transcendence of sexuality. Interestingly, while compelling queer narratives have been written critiquing childhood futurity, less queer scholarship has explored the queer temporalities and spatialities that accompany aging.[66] While the spatiality of the nursing home is conducive to desexualization and disposability, it need not be this way. The nursing home could be a space of community, communal living, alternate erotics, and life-sustaining relationships. In the following section, I explore how anti-ageist approaches seek to recuperate sexuality for aging adults, even while doing so through a dismissal of asexual possibilities.

## CHALLENGING DESEXUALIZATION

Research on sexuality and aging tends to draw on sexological paradigms, "reduc[ing] sexuality to a book-keeping approach that concerns who is still having sex . . . and how often."[67] Similar to early studies of so-called lesbian bed death, which I analyzed in the second chapter, research on sexuality and aging tends to quantify (hetero)sexual activity rather than think about the emotions, relationships, or contexts behind it. Also, in seeking to disprove the "asexuality" of older adults, much, indeed, most research inadvertently situates asexuality in a pejorative way, as inherently damaging to older adult health and well-being. On parallel to debates within critical disability studies, which until recently have sought sex-positive affirmations of disability through the distancing of disability from asexuality, this literature on critical aging presents asexuality as overwhelmingly undesirable and harmful to older adults without engaging affirmatively asexual perspectives.[68] Understandably, this distancing of older adult sexuality from asexuality takes place as a means to combat the institutional and discursive desexualization of older adulthood.

As the previous chapter discussed in relation to childhood, desexualization often gets misnamed as asexuality, including in relation to older adult sexuality. It is true that this misnaming could be simply attributed to a lack of literacy and visibility around asexuality, or to the lack of cross-over between critical geriatric studies or studies of aging and a/sexuality studies, or even to the paucity of language available in wide circulation to depict the nuances of nonsexualities. Nonetheless, I want to argue that this misnaming does damage to asexuality while ineffectually portraying the structures of desexualization. Most obviously, and as I discussed in previous chapters, such a misnaming denies the possibility for positive asexual identification, making asexual identity improbable, unbelievable, and undesirable. The conflation of asexuality

and desexualization, from an asexual studies standpoint, misrenders asexuality as something pejorative, life-inhibiting, and damaging.

Second, the misnaming of desexualization as asexuality provides a cover
for the oppressive biopolitical banning of sex. When older adults' desexualization is framed as "asexuality," it is rendered incidental, an effect of changing bodies, erasing the active process of disposal that makes aging sexuality
impossible. As long as aging is understood in terms of asexuality and not
in terms of desexualization, we are incapable of grasping the ongoing violence many encounter upon aging, of which a denial of sexuality is just one
component.

As an example, Katherine Bradway and Renée Beard, in "'Don't Be Trying
to Box Folks In': Older Women's Sexuality" (2015), argue that

> despite sex being a significant desire and need that all humans share and
> experience throughout the life course, older adults' sexual expression is often
> ignored or ridiculed by younger members of society. . . . That is, our youth-
> centric society problematizes aging bodies, assuming that aging negates the
> interest in or ability to be sexual; therefore, medicalized contemporary social
> constructions of the aging body relegate older adults to a sick, inherently
> asexual role.[69]

Agreeing with the rhetorical thrust of the piece—namely, that the rendering of older adults as nonsexual is an exercise in an ageist investment in the
disposability of aging adulthood—an asexually attuned analysis nonetheless
disagrees with Bradway and Beard's upholding of compulsory sexuality as a
"desire and need that all humans share," rendering asexuality inconceivable
as a sexual identity, as well as with their ableist dismissal of the "sick" older
adult.[70] Indeed, Bradway and Beard flesh out an entanglement in which a lack
of sex and sexuality is aligned with being "sick," mutually reinforcing disability
and asexuality as undesirable. To say that older adults are "asexual," or even
that they play such a role, is to dismiss the processes and contexts of aging, in
which bodies lose their entitlement to sex and sexuality as they are increasingly understood as disposable. The arguments that need to be made are thus
not that aging adults are sexual, but rather that aging adults are desexualized,
banned from their sexualities and from sex.

Similarly, some research tends to assert that sex and sexuality are necessarily healthy, discounting both the iterations of sex that may be deleterious,
including sex without consent, as well as possibilities for asexual aging. For
instance, as Emily Waterman writes in her study of college students' reac-

tions to the sexuality of older people, "research shows that a healthy sex life in old age greatly contributes to happiness and quality of life [. . . and that] premature loss of sexual functioning can contribute to emotional and physical deterioration in people; hanging onto sexuality can lessen feelings of loss in old age and increase self-esteem."[71] Such a conclusive statement, that sexuality and sex are necessarily healthful and that they can fight the harmful effects of aging, draws on compulsory sexuality to advocate for an extension of able-bodied healthiness into older age. Not only are possibilities for asexual aging edited out, but sex is encouraged at any cost—under what Simpson et al. call a "book-keeping approach" to sex that focuses only on how much, and mostly on heterosexual terms.[72] Such an approach to aging, which announces that if you have sex, you will stave off the effects of aging, disregards the social and biopolitical conditions under which aging bodies are rendered disposable.

This new "successful aging" paradigm includes the expansion of an ethics of optimism, bodily optimization, attractiveness, sexiness, health, vitality, and an active sex life to older segments of the population. While encouraging aging adults to remain active and "healthy" and to ward off isolation, such an approach tends to individualize aging, neglecting to account for the systemic disposability and ageism that aging bodies experience. It also does not conceive of survival as in itself a "success," neglecting the realities of racism, which makes survival into old age an accomplishment for those faced with racism in its many guises. In this account, it is active, quantifiable sex and sexual desire that become signals of "successful" and "healthy" aging.[73]

For example, Viagra, Flibanserin, hormone replacement, and other modes of sexual optimization have transformed what it means to have sex while aging, while binding sex to expert knowledge, access to pharmaceuticals, and upper-middle-class whiteness.[74] Treatments for sexual dysfunctions are meant to "reanimate [the] bodies and lives" of aging adults even while they consistently overlook queer and trans bodies.[75] In this sense, more and more older adults—of certain health, resources, ability, and vitality levels—are encouraged to engage in sex, seemingly undermining my argument that older adults are desexualized. Yet as Stephen Katz and Barbara Marshall suggest, such techniques of successful aging produce new norms for what it means to age, norms that are tightly tied to able-bodiedness and health as the new morality, as well as to wealth, couple privilege, and compulsory sexuality.[76] So while sex and sexuality are encouraged for some aging adults, this process is actually productive of a more stringent set of criteria for sexual citizenship, under which failure is imminent and self-monitoring is encouraged.[77] "Successful aging" thus emerges on particular terms that are not only compulsorily sexual, but also set against an imagined "bad aging" that is characterized by disability and ill health, or the "relentless hostility to physical decline and its tendency to regard health as a form of secular salvation."[78] Even the fit aging body is in need of self-surveillance so that it does not slip into symptoms of hated aging, which include slowness, inactivity, isolation, illness, and disability. Sexual activeness is part of this refusal to slow down, understood as functioning to ward away isolation, social decline, and overall bodily deterioration.

Notably, sexual fitness is also aestheticized, requiring particular gendered enactments of attractiveness, or "sexiness" throughout the life course that are difficult, expensive, and hazardous to maintain.[79] With the reconceptualization of "healthy" aging as a time of compulsory sexuality, desire disorders and physiological problems that are understood to get in the way of sex, including "'erectile dysfunction' [are framed] as a threat to both the physical and psychological well-being of an ageing population, and hence as a matter for public concern."[80] Critics of "successful aging" have thus argued that "the stereotype of the asexual old age" has "the potential to create a new myth about ageing sexuality, which is just as oppressive to older people as the stereotype it seeks to deconstruct"—entrenching sex as mandatory at all costs.[81] In refuting the "asexuality" of older adults, sex, sexiness, and sexual desire are produced as compulsory components of successful—that is, healthy, able-bodied, and responsible—aging, which is imbued with the potential to "stave off old age."[82] As compulsory sexuality is extended into older age, not only is the possibility for affirmative nonsexualities diminished, but the effects of desexualization—that is, of exclusion from the sexual fold—become more and more detrimental. Sex in older adult life thus becomes also a marker of a certain nondisposability among those lucky enough to retain access to it.

Some scholars discuss the ways in which aging sexuality provides insight on "the warmth and tenderness of emotional intimacy" or "the creation of a profound connection with another human while being acutely aware of one's own sense of wholeness as a separate person."[83] Affirming sexuality among older adults can thus also mean broadening notions of intimacy so that they include both touch- and non-touch-based connection, "the need for someone to be available to talk with and be close to; the need to be touched and appreciated, the need to smile, and the need to know someone else cares."[84] Celebrating aging adult sexuality could also shift strict understandings of sex to other forms of romantic touching, including cuddling, kissing, embracing, holding hands, and grooming, as well as solitary acts such as masturbation.[85] In this sense, aging in itself might present asexually attuned opportunities to question what constitutes desire and intimacy.

It is thus not that aging adults are not sexual, but rather that aging adults are produced as not sexual by ageist social structures. This production of desexualization is grounded in ideas that continue to inform white maturity as a site of an asexual ideal—that is, as a moral position of sexual distancing that characterizes the supreme evolutionary achievement of whiteness. The maturity narrative of asexuality—as both an evolutionary narrative of refined whiteness as sexually restrained as well as the narrative life arc as one ending in sexual disinterest—is used in turn to justify the enforcement of desexualization. This shift of focus I am suggesting is from understanding sexual decline as attributable to bodily senescence and deterioration to understanding sexual decline as a product of social fabrication stemming from an unjust corporeal politics. When research upholds asexual identification as undesirable for older adults, it tends to reinforce ideas that sex (especially for able-bodied aging adults) is either healthful or youth-maintaining. It also assumes that to be without sex is to be without erotic stimulation and to be less fulfilled, less of a person, and less of a "successful" ager. In the following section, I turn to an asexually affirmative analysis of older adulthood through exploring possibilities for spinsterly affectations and identifications. I draw forth possibilities for different models of aging that remain intent on cultivating erotics while being critical of compulsory sexuality.

## SPINSTERLY EROTICS

I shall close with a fantasy I have about these women, my neighbors in a huge and faceless 1950s high-rise that, like so many other such buildings with similar populations, stands like a sentinel on Chicago's northerly lakefront. My fantasy would offend them deeply but I think it unlikely that any will ever learn of it. While these women have made a sort of society for one another, each lives alone; I believe that many are lonely in the way one is lonely who has friends, but lacks a certain kind of intimacy. I believe too that many have what I called earlier "skin hunger." Here is my fantasy: these elderly widows abandon their deeply entrenched homophobia . . . and, just as they have learned to meet each other's needs for visibility and admiration, they go one step further and begin to meet each other's needs for physical intimacy. This intimacy need not be sexual, but if it is sexual, so much the better. Perhaps there are women whose needs extend farther than hugging and embracing, frequent nuzzling kisses, the comfort of a warm body touching one's own body in bed on a winter night. For the women who need sex and have not had it for decades, I fantasize wild sexual excitement and fulfillment and the special kind of confidence that comes with the knowledge that one has the capacity to arouse sexual desire in another. Their condo would come alive with couplings and rumors of couplings, dalliance, flirting, gossip, matchmaking, lovers' quarrels, *liaisons innocentes ou dangereuses*. Now these suddenly energetic sisters will have more to talk about than the ingratitude of their children, the day's ration of soap operas, or the thoroughly exhausted topic of the cuteness of their grandchildren.[86]

Michael Warner writes evocatively of all the relational forms that emerge from queer cultures: "each relation is an adventure in nearly uncharted territory. . . . There are almost as many types of relationships as there are people in combination. . . . Most have no labels. Most receive no public recognition. . . . Who among us would give them up?"[87] Widely read feminist theorist, Sandra Lee Bartky, in an essay titled "Unplanned Obsolescence: Some Reflections on Aging" (2000) offers us such a queerly potent, asexually resonant relational model of aging.[88] Speaking against the deadening and flattening landscape of "a huge and faceless 1950s high-rise," she envisions a utopian lesbian community of widows who fight the structural oppression of ageism by coming together to cultivate new forms of erotics.[89] Maintaining their spinsterly independence, the widows of this fantasy turn to each other for pleasure, solace, love, friendship, and what Bartky speaks of as "dalliance."[90]

There is much I am drawn to in this fantasy: widows coming together to discover the world anew through a lesbian utopia that confronts the structures of ageism, misogyny, couple privilege, and age-based segregation. Most of all, I am drawn to this fantasy for its capacity to speak affirmatively of aging adult sexuality even while deemphasizing sex on specific terms, and envisioning opportunities for asexual kinship, whether romantic or aromantic. As Bartky writes, "this intimacy need not be sexual" and includes "hugging and embracing, frequent nuzzling kisses, the comfort of a warm body touching one's own body in bed on a winter night," even while it also articulates "wild sexual excitement."[91] In short, Bartky's fantasy successfully frames an old age sex positivity that does not rely on compulsory sexuality or shut the door on asexuality.

In this section, I will explore an asexual aging that I wish to frame as spinsterly in disposition. I see this disposition as framed not around erotic absence but around erotic excess, and in excess of both lesbian and heterosexual identity categories. The spinster, a solitary figure on the edge of compulsory heterosexuality, heterosexual pair-bonding, the family nucleus, and the ritual of marriage, has appealed to many feminists, especially of the 1970s and 1980s, as a symbol of feminist refusal. She comes to stand in as well as a symbol of exclusion from the bounty of white society, even as she is white herself, providing insight into the excess that heteronormative power structures produce.

Most recently, modes of spinstering have begun to creep up in the main-stream, as is visible with Kate Bolick's ode to lavish and white middle-class singlehood, *Spinster: Making a Life of One's Own* (2015), as well as numerous popular articles that celebrate the term as an empowerment of women's single-hood.[92] A whole host of feminist recuperative readings of the spinster from the 1970s and 1980s set up the spinster as a feminist model of heterosexual refusal and lesbian resonance in times of patriarchal oppression.[93] For instance, Mary Daly in *Gyn/Ecology* (1978) spoke against the misogynist rendering of the spinster as lonely, old, and haggardly, remaking her as "she who has chosen her Self, who defines her Self, by choice, neither in relation to children nor to men, who is Self-identified, is a Spinster, a whirling dervish, spinning in a new time/space."[94] Similarly, Adrienne Rich has written of the spinster as engaged in "marriage resistance" as part of her lesbian continuum that talks back to compulsory heterosexuality.

Historians and literary scholars have sought to temper this celebratory reading of the spinster by drawing attention to the realities and representa-tions of the spinster historically.[95] In *Never Married*, Amy Froide demonstrates that historically, and specifically between 1550 and 1750, marital status was a fundamental "category of difference" in England, a distinction as significant as class would have been, even while married adults have been the focus of most historical research.[96] The "spinster," Froide outlines, was used to describe women of various ages, from early girlhood until old age, and large segments of women remained "never married" or "singlewomen"—up to 30 percent, depending on the town and period. Spinsters were not always isolated but were frequently woven into the fabric of their communities and kin networks. While the meaning of the term "spinster" was initially a woman who spun as her occupation, the pejorative use of the term arose in the later seventeenth century, at which point never-married women were "satirized, scorned, and . . . derided as a menace to English society."[97]

Kathryn Kent, exploring literary representations in the nineteenth- and early twentieth-century US, argues that the development of the spinster iden-tity coincided with an increase in white unmarried women caused by the death of men in the US Civil War. As a "protolesbian" identity resonant with queer and feminine modes of relating and abstaining from heterosexuality, spinsterhood both made women vulnerable to "the whims of their brothers and fathers" and created spaces for new subjectivities to form with increased access to education and the public realm.[98] Spinsterhood usually refers to white women, Kent argues, because single status or refusal to marry carried different meanings for African American women than it did for white women. While white middle-class women were increasingly seeking inclusion in the public sphere outside of marriage, marriage itself was a means for African American women to enter public life, drawing on Hortense Spillers.[99] Spinsterhood thus emerged as an identity attached to whiteness, and as at odds, in certain ways, with "proper" heterosexual coupling and reproduction.

Interestingly, while the spinster can easily be associated with lacking a partner, she has also signified historically as a figure of excess—both economic and sexual, as a counterpoint and extension of bourgeois maternity unfettered by heterosexual marriage.[100] Kent writes of the spinster as a figure of the "excess and extraness" of erotic energy unchanneled into heterosexual partnering.[101] The white spinster in Victorian colonial contexts was considered "superfluous," as "surplus," and "redundant" until she was repackaged as a national commodity for use in nation building, as Rita Kranidis describes.[102] Similarly, the female schoolteacher, often a spinster, "came to signify 'sexual abnormality' (lesbian as opposed to mere abstinence)" that was tied to social anxieties about gendered norms and proper heterosexual behavior.[103] Thus while the spinster is easily understood as a figure of sexual lack, she is also a figure of excess. This excess is twofold: suggesting an excess of erotic energies that results in the burgeoning of ulterior modes of relating and a mode of identity that is not reducible to either heterosexuality or lesbian identification.

The spinster, a feminist specter of bygone days, comprises an asexually resonant refusal to be disposable, by refusing—by circumstance or strategy—to attach to heteronormative life cycles, time orders, and compulsory sexuality. While the couple is an integral institution of social organization and sociality, it works to manufacture some people as surplus and excess.[104] Caleb Luna writes that being *singled* in a context where others are coupled is to have care and investment withdrawn from you, to be "denied intimacy and care from those in my life, who reserve it for others."[105] Couple privilege is such that life is easier to negotiate at the financial and pragmatic levels when in a couple, for the simple reason that society is designed with the couple in mind.[106] Coupling offers a framework for how love, care, attentiveness, and desire are to be shared along gendered lines. And coupling is nothing if not the making of citizenship units intended as the building blocks of a nation, a society, and thus buoyed along by structural support.[107] Marital and couple frameworks are also a form of settler colonial order, implemented to the effect of eradicating kinship structures and their role in sovereign modes of governance among Indigenous people.[108] The spinster, as a white figure of excess that has slipped out of the governing structure of couplehood, is a figure of both loneliness and erotic possibility. Loneliness or joy are not here mutually exclusive experiences but ones that are entangled in each other. While, as Heather Love explores, loneliness is central to queer experiences of the spinster under conditions of coupled patriarchy, joy consists of those queer relatings that Warner explores—unsanctioned, unrecognized, but thickly real and intimate.[109] The figure of the spinster surfaces as a figure of radical refusal and excessive erotics and relatings that responds to the limits of couple formation and the ways they exclude anyone who is not in the care and attention that a coupled life purports to provide.

Second, the spinster figures as in excess of heterosexual and lesbian identification, arising as an asexually resonant identity distinct from other identities. Drawing on Benjamin Kahan, the spinster's "solitude [is] a mode of relation. Solitary existence is not the isolating loneliness of the closet but rather a fully contented mode of sociability."[110] Drawing on Kahan's work on celibacy, spinsterly life-modes are not substitutes for lesbian identification or terms of closeting but distinct and articulate modes of living life. In this sense, while the spinster has a distinct historical lineage as an identity category, contemporary forms of spinstering may be akin to what Peter Coviello discusses as "competing conceptions of the very *domain* of sexuality," erotic modes not encompassable by the terms available under rubrics of sexual identification.[111] The spinster is thus a figure with both a historical lineage and one that slips out of, erotically, the terms of identification available today.

In mining the figure of the spinster, I am interested in both the loneliness and joy that spinsterly erotics facilitate: the experiences of desexualization and being singled (rendered unlovable by society) as well as of queer world-making and erotic possibility. In mobilizing around the figure of the spinster, I am interested in the way it speaks in multiple voices: as a queer asexually resonant figure who is exemplary of a life lived otherwise, as someone who draws our attention to the structures of the couple as a site of privilege, as an opening up onto structural critiques of aging and disposability, and as a figure of excessive erotics.[112] Crucially, I see the spinster as affiliated with aging womanhood but not defined by it, since as a "figure [they are] intensely fluid."[113]

The spinster might present an opening here for a queer and asexually attuned model of aging that wrestles with disposability but does not give in to demands to prove worth, health, vitality, or liveliness through sexual participation. In this sense, I see spinsterhood as in dissonance with the couple formation, a call to the alternate rhythms of life. The spinster might find joy in that sort of sensuality not easily classifiable as "sex"—a sensuality not quantifiable, a making do with life, and a reaching out to the world in search of spinsterly companions. If queer scholars have commented on "sideways" growth and "extended adolescence," is it not possible that spinstral aging offers its own rhythms of space and time relations?[114] Spinstral time, then, is a time that spirals, that coils against itself, suspicious of couple privilege and the misogynist and ableist structures of ageism and old-age disposability. Spinstrality is a spinning of the self, a refusal of activity and productivity that is nonetheless creative, in the sense that it prioritizes queer and asexual modes of relating and inventing the self against structures that seek to demolish it. As my next section will explore by drawing on the figure of *Frances Ha* in the film by the same name, a spinsterly disposition involves an asexual erotics of excess.

## SPINSTERLY EXCESS IN *FRANCES HA*

One of the most spinsterly accounts of erotics I have encountered is in the mumblecore film *Frances Ha* (2012), directed by Noah Baumbach and written by Baumbach and Greta Gerwig. Mumblecore is a genre obsessed with whiteness and its accompanying affects in contemporary contexts, such as restlessness, boredom, and a perceived loss of entitlement. Deploying dry wit, mumblecore is characterized less by plot lines than by tracking the erotics or miserotics of relationships.[115] As a film on white subjectivity, *Frances Ha* offers insight into erotics, whiteness, and their entanglement, through the spinsterly excessive figure of Frances Ha.

*Frances Ha,* as I will offer, presents a way to imagine an asexual erotics that verges on queer asexual spinsterhood, and that is rife with "styles of erotic being that may not rise to the level of 'discourse.'"[116] *Frances Ha,* I suggest, hints at erotic tendencies that are not dilutable to lesbian, straight, bi, or poly identification, but that tingle with an asexual mode of erotic relating that is in excess of present-day identity categories and life rhythms. Drawing on Coviello's work, which engages with the histories of erotic formation prior to the sexual signification system we are familiar with, *Frances Ha* is full of "spaces of lag, delay, and suspension . . . a variety of styles of erotic being and their [struggle to become] legible as *form*."[117] The film also showcases the white spinsterly character of Frances as herself a figure of excess, and one not easily made compliant to straight modes of love and work. Throughout the film, attracting is rendered as not strictly sexual but rather suggestive of an asexual erotics that are not containable by any identity category, dreaming of alternative ways in which intimacies, friendships, and erotics can take form as well as of the loneliness and joy intrinsic to spinstering.[118] Crucially, what we learn about asexuality from *Frances Ha* is that attraction can and does exist on not strictly sexual but erotic terms and that asexual attracting can be a queer challenge to reproductive orders. Asexuality emerges less an as ideal of whiteness than as a mode of undesirable excess, loneliness, and inability to transform one's life according to the American Dream of success.

In *Frances Ha,* Frances Halladay (Greta Gerwig), the white protagonist, is a figure rendered both lovable and lost. For most of the film she lingers in a depressed, stretched present of no money, no job prospects, and no sexual relationships on the horizon. Given that her very best friend (also white), who is "basically the same person as her but with different hair," moves out of their joint apartment in New York at the beginning of the film, Frances is itinerant, taking up residence with one acquaintance and then another, trying to warm a place for herself as a single (spinster) woman in other people's lives without resorting to sexual coupling.[119] Tragically, Frances is deeply and devotedly in love with her best friend, a rather self-oriented and heteronormatively bound Sophie (Mickey Sumner). When we first meet Frances and Sophie, they are "like a lesbian couple that doesn't have sex anymore" since they spend all their nonwork hours together: smoking on the parapet, sleeping in the same bed, play fighting in the park, and declaring their love to one another.[120] The two even have a future-bound origin story, a "story of us" that Frances likes to hear as an incantation of a possible life shared with her very closest companion. Frances loves Sophie despite their clear lack of sexual attraction, and despite Sophie "lov[ing] [her] phone that has email more than [her]."[121] As the door of her youth closes and as Frances enters the space of spinsterhood, she learns to accept that she will not be Sophie's life companion but only her "three hour brunch friend," learning at the same time to enter the world of straight time: acquiring a low-paying but more full-time desk job at the company she danced for as an apprentice, renting her own apartment, and finally, through placing her name—or whatever fits of it ("Frances Ha")—on her mailbox.[122] Yet even while she succumbs to the straight facts of life, Frances's asexual love for and unnamable erotic draw to Sophie lingers.

From love, Frances wants

> this one moment . . . which might explain why I'm still single . . . It's that thing when you're with someone and you love them and they know it and they love you and you know it but it's a party and you're both talking to other people and you're laughing and shining and you look across the room and catch each others' eyes but not because you're possessive or it's precisely sexual but because that is your person in this life and it's funny and sad but only because this life will end and it's the secret world that exists right there in public, unnoticed that no one else knows about . . . That's what I want out of a relationship.[123]

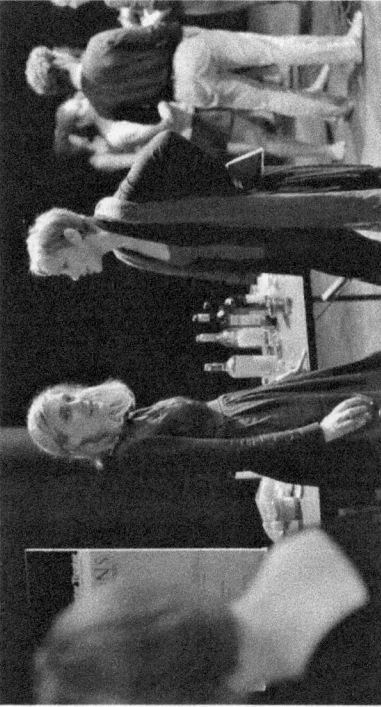

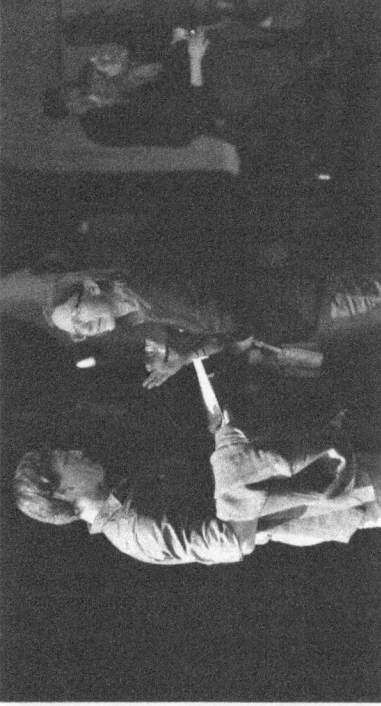

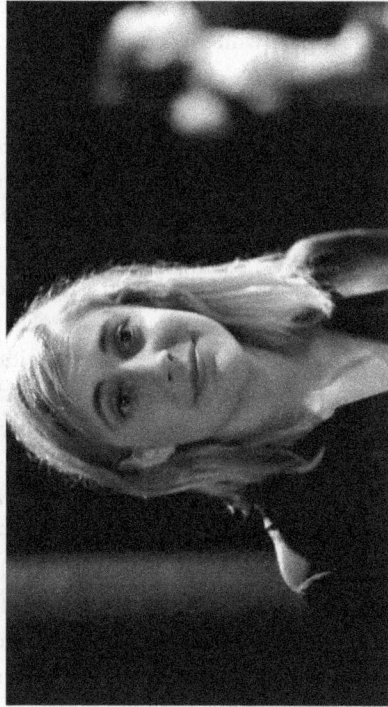

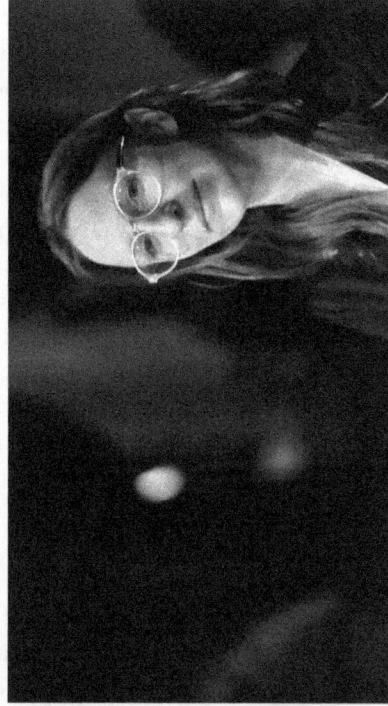

**FIGURE 4.1.** Frances (left) and Sophie (right) gaze at each other in public. Stills from *Frances Ha*, 2012.

It is not surprising, then, that in the very last minutes of the film, just as Frances's life is falling into place and she begins to succumb to her lonely spinsterly lot in life as a secretary who dances on the side, Frances experiences this moment of great intimacy that is not "possessive" or "precisely sexual" with Sophie (see figure 4.1). Frances sees Sophie, and perhaps for the first time, Sophie sees Frances back, in a crowded room, shortly after a dance performance that Frances has curated. Seeing here is a moment of being with the other and indulging in that togetherness—it is, in short, what we are taught the sex act, especially the sex act with "simultaneous orgasm," is supposed to be.[124] It is a moment that questions what sex and sexuality could be, "friendly but not chaste," erotically charged.[125] They see each other, and they are moved by this moment of seeing each other—across a room, segmented into different life spaces and times, but together, in a moment of romantic asexual attracting. Frances's perseverant asexual love for Sophie illustrates the queer and erotic capacities of asexuality.

Their erotic moment of gazing at each other, which viewers are invited to behold, provides a moment of the gaze as recognition as well as separation. The gaze has been theorized as a central forum through which the self learns of the other. For instance, Jacques Lacan proposed the gaze as a major step in subject formation, of recognizing oneself in the mirror as an entity apart and unique from others, and Frantz Fanon established the white gaze as a way through which whiteness establishes itself as superior.[126] On one level, Sophie and Frances's gaze challenges these theories of the gaze as separation since it is only in this moment of gazing at each other that Sophie can recognize Frances and take her as she is and that Frances achieves the erotic satisfaction she has been seeking from her best friend throughout the film. Frances, in short, both sees and is seen in this moment. On the other hand, Sophie, as successfully white, and Frances, as faltering in her capacity to project the good life of whiteness, cannot hold their gaze of recognition for long. Their gaze, while intensely, asexually erotic, is a gaze that can only unify them momentarily as life continues to flow along its individualized and heteronormative routes. Throughout the film, whiteness is not challenged as a position of neutrality, nor is a critical gaze to whiteness cultivated among audiences as the cast of characters is presented merely as diverse individuals rather than as variations of whiteness struggling to achieve the promises of the good life white middle-classness is supposed to provide.[127] Yet Frances emerges as a figure of excess, entangled in projects of whiteness but also in excess of them.

Frances Ha's romantic asexual affliction for her best friend Sophie is but one constitutive element of her queer and untimely spinster persona. She is a figure of excess. Frances's asexual perversion—her great asexual love for her best friend—exists alongside her inability and unwillingness to conform to a life that encourages the channeling of desires into work under a capitalist order, into love in a reproductive order, and into the maintenance of an atomistic self buttressed by the hetero-coupled formation. While these markers of the "good life" are indeed fraying, as Lauren Berlant extrapolated, their fantasy still holds space in the social order.[128] Whiteness, in turn, shores up as a racist practice for guarding against the perceived loss of entitlement and bounty. With some vestiges of white middle-class privilege, Frances struggles against succumbing to heteronormative rhythms but is drawn, despite herself, into a straight time and an expanded precarious now that is not working up to any projected, improved future. Frances, with her inability to get out, network, build projects, and with her tired attitude to the thinness of sociality under late capitalism—where a best friend becomes, overnight, a "three hour brunch friend"—ultimately fails at reproducing a chrononormative straight time.[129] She is more inclined to being itinerant, dancing in the streets, and overflowing with emotion than securing a sexual partnership or work-life balance. In her spinsterly disposition, she fails at being included into the warm glow of coupled culture. Frances, dallying her way through the city's streets and through her life course, demonstrates a failed approach to heteronormative success that is akin to the spinsters that feminist historians and literary scholars draw out from the archives. She exists as the excess and debris of whiteness—both white and superfluous to the projects of aspirational white, college-educated youth, which her friends are ardently upkeeping. To use Sara Ahmed's language, Frances is orientated "slantwise" away from what is supposed to matter and toward the indefinable serendipity of life.[130] Frances's desires are channeled slantwise through the apparatus of attraction, as she is attracted not so much sexually as asexually. Her asexual attractions hint at an asexual erotics that are defiant of the common sexual track and its coexistence with heteronormativity, coitality, and chrononormativity.

Frances Ha is suggestive of a spinsterly asexual erotics of excess that reverberates through the psychic life of the protagonist. These erotics, crucially, are a queerly asexual sensation, in that they provide an erotic relational challenge to dominant, straight ways of life structuring. Frances's aexual erotics challenge the sexual imperative of compulsory sexuality and the idea that happiness and the good life are maintained through sexual relating. Attraction here does not function to channel the protagonist along heterosexual or sexual lines, but rather along asexual slants. Intimacy is formed, erotically, through a different, "slantwise" or unintelligible form of attraction.[131] It is not that Frances challenges whiteness but that she is lost when it comes to upholding it or reaping its many privileges because she is in spinsterly excess of its coupled structures. *Frances Ha*'s asexual erotics are that of a romantic lesbian friendship, a spinster-sisterhood, Boston marriage, or those "lesbian relationships that are romantic and erotic, but that don't include sexual activity."[132] Yet, interestingly, Frances does not surface as "a lesbian" in the film, nor is her sexual orientation or gender confirmed by the directional pull of her asexual attraction. She remains unbound by sexual identities, yet highly amative—that is, disposed to being loving, amorous. This, of course, suggests an inadequacy in identificatory naming rituals. Similarly, it hints at the failure in recent years for "lesbian" to hold space for asexual erotics as well as the irreducibility of sexual identity to sexual attraction. While a figure of spinstral excess and asexual attracting, Frances's love, life, and modes of relating are ultimately erratic and irreducible to any one identity. Through both joy and loneliness, the spinsterly Frances of *Frances Ha* provides a compelling representation of erotic models of aging that are asexually resonant, erotically charged, and in excess of modes and models of sexual identification. The spinster offers another avenue for thinking about asexual erotics as not lacking but as potentially excessive of capitalistic white structures, identity categories, and contemporary modes of being together.

## THE QUEER ASEXUALITY OF AGING

As Shannon Bell has written: "It doesn't matter how many years one has worked out, or how long and hard each time, time will get you."[133] As a queer feminist still touching youth and mimicking its aesthetics and implorations, I often slip into a disbelief of aging. While entering old age might still feel distant for me at an embodied level, I need only to look at my own family's line of aging matriarchs to be reminded of the body's proneness to age. Spinsterhood, as I have considered throughout this chapter, offers a fluid category with which to think queer aging on terms that make sense of both the isolation of living on queer terms and the joy that fecund moments of erotic relating provide. In these ways, spinsterhood offers an alternative model to fighting desexualization and disposability than sexual celebration, asking that we remain open to asexual erotics.

# EPILOGUE

# Tyrannical Celibacy

## *The Anti-Erotics of Misogyny and White Supremacy*

AS I WAS completing work on this book, a tyrannical event befell my beloved city of Toronto, Ontario, which forced me to reckon with the dangerous possibilities of nonsexuality and the limits of projects for an erotic rethinking of sexuality. On April 23, 2018, Alek Minassian, a self-declared "incel," or someone who is involuntarily celibate, drove a van on the sidewalks of the bustling Yonge Street and Finch Avenue intersection and down Yonge Street's sidewalks through to Sheppard Avenue with the intent of plowing over as many pedestrians as possible. Killing ten and injuring sixteen people, he was apprehended by the police, yet the white Minassian himself suffered no injuries from the attack or the police, a testimony to the protection whiteness can offer even to the most tyrannical of attackers. While people of all genders were injured, information quickly leaked out that the attack was misogynist in nature, inspired by Minassian's feelings of having been denied sex by women and his subsequent identification as an incel, an involuntarily celibate. Information also transpired that Minassian was inspired by Elliot Rodger, who in 2014 undertook a mass shooting targeting women at a sorority house at a university in California. Rodger shot at the "Chads and Stacys," or, respectively, those men who received sex and those women who denied him sex.[1] Minassian, Rodger, and others congregate in the dark corners of the internet, such as at Incel.me and Reddit forums, and plan, both symbolically and materially, of organizing "incel rebellions" that include taking down a system in which women can deny sex to men and in which some men receive more access to sex with women than others.[2]

To detractors of asexuality, it would not be a far leap to conflate the sexual identity with the tyrannical celibacy of the incels. Yet, as I hope is clear, these communities have nothing to do with each other. Asexuality is widely understood as a sexual orientation that does not, in most cases, mourn the loss of sex or sexual desire and that more broadly challenges us to unthink our attachments to compulsory sexuality, or, as this book has explored, the idea that sex and sexual desire are presumed to be natural, innate, and consistent for all people, and most especially for white, heterosexual, able-bodied, and coupled individuals. At the most basic level, on the other hand, involuntary celibacy suggests the reverse—that if one is not provided sex or is denied sex, one is incomplete, unfulfilled, and lacking. Incel rhetoric speaks acutely to the existence of compulsory sexuality as a system that presumes that everyone is sexual—that is, desiring of sex—and it also fortifies tyrannical forms of hatred in which, as Minassian and Rodger evince, some white cisgender heterosexual men assume they are entitled to an endless flow of sex from women.

What does it mean that men can feel so enraged by not being provided sex from women that they will kill others and themselves to take a political stance against this denial? I would suggest that this speaks, first, to the entrenchment of compulsory sexuality in systems of misogyny, the very same misogyny that feminists of the late 1960s and 1970s set out to dismantle with their theorizations and applications of political asexuality, as I analyzed in the first chapter. Feminists and feminist groups such as Cell 16, the Young Lords Party, Toni Cade Bambara, Valerie Solanas, The Feminists, and The Furies, while articulating varying visions of political asexuality/celibacy in the context of the 1960s and 1970s, each responded to the oppressive conditions of heteropatriarchy under which sex was understood as a good that women give to men, and that men are entitled to receive from women. In such a system, compulsory sexuality is not only the celebration of sex or sexual desire but it is the uneven application of this celebration—the idea that white men *deserve* sex and women owe them this sex. In their foundational understandings of compulsory sexuality, these feminists, across social locations and political projects, all provided a deep critique of compulsory sexuality as a system within which gender is supported on very narrow binary terms that function to consistently disadvantage women through this understanding that men are entitled to women. It was thus that projects of political celibacy/asexuality made sense, because through refusing to abide by the expectations of a gender system in which women *owed* men sex, women cultivated different forms of communities, self-knowledge, and political projects. Ever since I began reading these early critiques of compulsory sexuality, I have been enamored by this feminist willfulness to say no as an erotic mode of world transformation in itself.

The Minassians and Rodgers, on the other hand, reflect their own tyrannical rebellion that is fuelled by rage at feminist projects of refusal and their legacies for rethinking the centrality of sex and injustice. For while perhaps compulsory sexuality has arguably intensified as sex has become increasingly tied to notions of health, wellness, and fulfillment, sex has also provided possibilities for challenging gender binaries, couple culture, and heteronormativity. And yet, is it not also telling that a denial of sex continues to wound white heterosexual (and cisgender) masculinity? Minassian and Rodger felt, literally, wounded by not being able to extract sex from women. In this sense, it seems that a denial of sex led to a crisis of white masculinity, which fueled tyrannical rage, suggesting that compulsory sexuality is bound not only to ideas of men being able to expect sex from women but also to whiteness and ideas of white entitlement to have a life that includes abundant sex. Further still, it is only within a social context of compulsory sexuality that masculinity can feel wounded by not receiving sex. If sex was not understood as an indelible right, and an indelible right for white men in particular, then an absence of sex would not be experienced as a wounding and incel rage on these terms would not be conceivable.

Incel reminds us of the ways in which white masculinity, in particular, is wounded when it is denied what has been assumed for too long to be a birthright: domination, supremacy, access to other bodies for the fulfillment of one's own erotics. Casey Ryan Kelly explores Elliot Rodger's 140-page tome titled "My Twisted World," a manifesto of white patriarchal supremacy grounded in affects of anger and loneliness.[3] Without discussing the manuscript in great length, I want to demonstrate the way in which it speaks to the intersection of white supremacy, compulsory sexuality, and misogyny. In it Rodger discusses his feelings of entitlement to women, his surprise at not being desired by them and gaining access to them, as well as his racist outrage that a black acquaintance is sexually successful when he is not. Rodger writes, "How could an inferior, ugly black boy be able to get a white girl and not me? I am beautiful, and I am half white myself. I am descended from British aristocracy. He is descended from slaves."[4] In this tyrannical disposition, Rodger mourns the way in which his imagined birthright of white supremacy is not fully realized because he has been denied sex by women. The girl his acquaintance loses his virginity to is a white blond girl, furthering Rodger's fury. Speaking to the entanglement of compulsory sex with sexism and racism, Rodger expresses outrage at not having sex flowing in his direction, expressing his deep sense of being entitled to women's bodies and also black bodies through recalling practices of enslavement. In recalling slavery, he sees it as speaking to the worthlessness of blackness instead of the tyranny of whiteness, exonerating whiteness as a site of purity, good breeding, and fitness to rule. Rodger ends his journal planning a "Day of Retribution" as a form of punishing men who receive pleasure from women and women who deny him his birthright of pleasure. He also spares time to flesh out his deep misogyny of women as "the ultimate evil . . . beasts . . . a plague" who should not be able to "choose who to mate and breed with," have rights, and be instead "quarantine[d] . . . in concentration camps" as well as eradicated.[5] Both Minassian's and Rodger's attacks speak to but one example of the rage that is ignited when white masculinity is denied unencumbered supremacy. It is also, importantly, rooted in a colonial, white, patriarchal culture that at every turn—for centuries—has validated men's access to women, and white access to bodies of color.[6]

I want to return now to Audre Lorde's formulation of the erotic through which this book is structured.[7] Lorde, we can recall, positioned the erotic as a powerful source for addressing racism and sexism and as an energy that women can access toward leading more full and self-determined lives, even within contexts of patriarchy. The erotic provides strength and fuel for living a life of self-determination and satisfaction, and for challenging racism and sexism at the deepest level. Lorde also warned, however, of misusing the erotic, of using one's own desire for being erotically fulfilled toward the destruction of others. To rob another of the capacity of the erotic in pursuit of one's own erotic is for Lorde a grave dysfunction characteristic of colonial, white, and sexist systems that treat bodies and sex as commodities to be owned. We can understand the actions of Minassian and Rodger in such a context. Unable to find erotic self-fulfillment and life satisfaction, unable to reap fully the benefits they felt they were owed within white patriarchal supremacy, Minassian and Rodger unleash terror on others.

Further still, tyrannical celibacy speaks to the odd uses and misuses of political theories, concepts, and terms. "Incel" itself first emerged as a term coined in 1993 by a queer woman intent on analyzing restrictive gender norms rather than as an emblem of misogyny and the "manosphere" with which it is associated today.[8] On an even more disturbing level, much of Elliot Rodger's angry tract is reminiscent of some feminist work from the 1960s and 1970s, which advocated for an end to compulsory sexuality. Rodger assesses that it is through sex that women have too much power, drawing on the sexist undercurrents of compulsory sexuality to fuel his tyrannical misogyny. In his frustration with being denied sex, Rodger envisions a world in which no one will have sex, and "sexuality . . . must be outlawed." For, he continues, "in a world without sex, humanity will be pure and civilized," thus drawing on white discourses of purity and asexuality-as-ideal toward validating his misogyny.[9]

Reminiscent especially of Valerie Solanas, Rodger's words misunderstand injustice, making possible a reverse understanding of sexism and racism in the world as being directed against men and whiteness. In his text, Rodger claims frequently that he is experiencing "injustice" even while mentioning slavery or when providing misogynist and hateful language against women. Understanding injustice as a denial of birthright and entitlement of white men under whiteness and patriarchy, the concept of injustice becomes usurped from its antiracist and antisexist leanings toward serving to reestablish the validity of misogyny within white supremacy. The case of incel thus demonstrates how white supremacists and alt-right men can mobilize language of injury and victimhood, as well as saviorship, misreading the historically grounded legacies of injustice. Political celibacy/asexuality also becomes misused in tyrannical ways to justify misogyny and racism. Accidentally drawing on feminist political celibacy/asexuality, Rodger misattributes the injustice of the world to women because he experiences doubt over his white entitlement to bodies as unjust in itself. In these racist and sexist uses, "involuntary celibacy" emerges as an anti-erotic tool intent on speaking against feminist and antiracist progress, building a world within which white men can continue to have unfettered access to the bodies of others. If anything, incel-inspired tyranny demarcates the ways in which it is imperative that compulsory sexuality be analyzed as a site at which whiteness and patriarchy intersect. Erotics, in turn, inform the decentering of compulsory sexuality, challenging anti-erotic deployments of hatred.

*Asexual Erotics* is neither a definitive nor a complete exploration of what erotics, asexually conceived, might look like and how they might inflect our readings of compulsory sexuality. It is rather an exploration of capacious asexuality that struggles to wrest ideas of intimate relating as well as understandings of feminism, queerness, and lesbianism away from sex and sexual desire. Compulsory sexuality has deep effects that intersect with racism, sexism, and ableism and that permeate the functions of these systems. On the other hand, as this book has explored, feminism, queerness, and lesbianism are rife with moments of erotic relating that are not sexual in any self-evident way but that rather draw on various aspects of asexuality either as an explicit critique of compulsory sexuality or in more subtle ways as a mode of feeling and connection. These moments and forms of erotics, as I have been exploring, provide avenues for envisioning worlds in which compulsory sexuality is critiqued and undermined—as it must be if we are to undermine tyranny in its many forms.

# NOTES

## NOTES TO ACKNOWLEDGMENTS

1. Leah Lakshmi Piepzna-Samarasinha, *Bodymap: Poems* (Toronto: Mawenzi House, 2015), 41–42.


## NOTES TO INTRODUCTION

1. Cameron Awkward-Rich, "A Prude's Manifesto," *Button Poetry* 2015, https://www.facebook.com/ButtonPoetry/videos/1277265262331016/?hc_ref=PAGES_TIMELINE.
2. For an introduction to asexuality, see Angela Tucker's *(A)sexual* (New York City, Big Mouth Films, Arts Engine, 2011).
3. Adrienne Rich, "Compulsory Heterosexuality and Lesbian Existence," *Signs: Journal of Women in Culture and Society* 5, no. 4 (1980): 631–60. See Elizabeth F. Emens, "Compulsory Sexuality," *Stanford Law Review* 66, no. 2 (2014): 303–86 and Kristina Gupta, "Compulsory Sexuality: Evaluating an Emerging Concept," *Signs: Journal of Women in Culture and Society* 41, no. 1 (2015): 141.
4. Kathleen Stewart, *Ordinary Affects* (Durham, NC: Duke University Press, 2007), 3.
5. AVEN: Asexual Visibility and Education Network, 2001–2012, https://www.asexuality.org.
6. Eve Kosofsky Sedgwick, *Tendencies* (Durham, NC: Duke University Press, 1993), 8.
7. Audre Lorde, "Uses of the Erotic: The Erotic as Power" (1978), in *Sister Outsider*, 53–59 (Freedom, CA: The Crossing Press, 1984).
8. Bryce J. Renninger, "'Where I Can Be Myself . . . Where I Can Speak My Mind:' Networked Counterpublics in a Polymedia Environment," *New Media and Society* 17, no. 9 (2015): 1513–29.
9. Cole Brown, "The History of the Asexual Community," presented at *Asexual Countercultures: Exploring Ace Communities and Intimacies,* Vancouver, BC, Simon Fraser University, November 2, 2017; AVEN, https://www.asexuality.org.
10. Kristin S. Scherrer, "Coming to an Asexual Identity: Negotiating Identity, Negotiating Desire," *Sexualities* 11, no. 5 (2008): 621–41.
11. David Jay, *A Look at Online Collective Identity Formation,* May 13, 2003, 3–5. Andrew Hinderliter, *Asexuality: The History of a Definition | Asexual Explorations* (2009), http://www.asexualexplorations.net/home/history_of_definition.html; "The Haven for the

Human Amoeba," *Yahoo Groups,* http://groups.yahoo.com/group/havenforthehuman-amoeba/; Zoe O'Reilly, "My Life as an Amoeba," *StarNet Dispatches* (1997).

12. O'Reilly, "My Life as an Amoeba."

13. CJ DeLuzio Chasin, "Making Sense in and of the Asexual Community: Navigating Relationships and Identities in a Context of Resistance," *Journal of Community & Applied Social Psychology* 25, no. 2 (2015): 176.

14. Elizabeth Brake, *Minimizing Marriage: Marriage, Morality, and the Law* (Oxford: Oxford University Press, 2012), 90–102.

15. AVEN, https://www.asexuality.org/?q=general.html.

16. Sedgwick, *Tendencies,* 7.

17. Sedgwick, *Epistemology of the Closet* (Berkeley: University of California Press, 1990), 35.

18. Sedgwick, *Tendencies,* 7–9; Sedgwick, *Epistemology of the Closet,* 35.

19. Michel Foucault, *The History of Sexuality: An Introduction, Vol. I.,* trans. Robert Hurley (New York: Vintage Books, 1978/1990).

20. Ann Laura Stoler, *Race and the Education of Desire: Foucault's History of Sexuality and the Colonial Order of Things* (Durham, NC: Duke University Press, 1995).

21. Alfred C. Kinsey, Wardell B. Pomeroy, and Clyde E. Martin, *Sexual Behavior in the Human Male* (Philadelphia: W. B. Saunders, 1948).

22. Also see Avenwiki, "Lexicon," http://wiki.asexuality.org/Lexicon.

23. Maisha, *Taking the Cake: An Illustrated Primer on Asexuality* (2012): cover and page 10. Available for free download here: https://acezinearchive.files.wordpress.com/2015/01/taking_the_cake_-_double_sided_printing_fixed.pdf.

24. Julie Sondra Decker, *The Invisible Orientation: An Introduction to Asexuality* (New York City: Skyhorse Publishing, 2016), 88. Sedgwick, *Epistemology of the Closet,* 25–26.

25. Mary Kame Ginoza, Tristan Miller, and the AVEN Survey Team, *The 2014 AVEN Community Census: Preliminary Findings* (2014), https://asexualcensus.files.wordpress.com/2014/11/2014censuspreliminaryreport.pdf. Also see Asexual Awareness Week Team and Tristan Miller (aka Siggy), "Asexual Community Census 2011" (2011), http://asexualawarenessweek.comfdocsfSiggyAnalysis-AAWCensus.pdf.

26. Pádraig MacNeela and Aisling Murphy, "Freedom, Invisibility, and Community: A Qualitative Study of Self-Identification with Asexuality," *Archives of Sexual Behavior* 44, no. 3 (2015): 799.

27. Ginoza, Miller, and the AVEN Survey Team, *The 2014 AVEN Community Census.*

28. Eunjung Kim, "Asexualities and Disabilities in Constructing Sexual Normalcy," in *Asexualities: Feminist and Queer Perspectives,* ed. KJ Cerankowski and M. Milks (New York: Routledge, 2014); Cara C. MacInnis and Gordon Hodson, "'Intergroup Bias towards "Group X:' Evidence of Prejudice, Dehumanization, Avoidance, and Discrimination against Asexuals," *Group Processes and Intergroup Relations* 15, no. 6 (2012): 740.

29. MacNeela and Murphy, "Freedom, Invisibility, and Community."

30. Maisha, *Taking the Cake,* 7.

31. Chasin, "Making Sense in and of the Asexual Community," 174; A. K. Morrissey, "Remedial Asexuality: Sexualnormativity in Health Care," in *The Remedy: Queer and Trans Voices on Health and Health Care,* ed. Zena Sherman (Vancouver: Arsenal Pulp Press, 2016), 166–67, 173. Also see KJ Cerankowski, "Spectacular Asexuals: Media Visibility and Cultural Fetish," in *Asexualities: Feminist and Queer Perspectives,* ed. KJ Cerankowski and M. Milks (New York: Routledge, 2014); Ginoza, Miller, and the AVEN Survey Team, *The 2014 AVEN Community Census;* Ela Przybylo, "Masculine Doubt and Sexual Wonder: Asexually-Identified Men Talk about Their (A)sexualites," in *Asexualities: Feminist and Queer Perspectives,* ed. M. Milks and KJ Cerankowski (New York: Routledge, 2014).

32. Sebastian Grace, "What's R(ace) and RAD Got to Do with It? Musings of a Transracially Adopted Asexual," in *Brown and Gray,* ed. jnramos, 2015; Julian B. Carter, *The Heart of Whiteness: Normal Sexuality and Race in America, 1880–1940* (Durham, NC: Duke University Press, 2012). Also see Ianna Hawkins Owen, "Still, Nothing: Mammy and Black Asexual Possibility," *Feminist Review* 120, no. 1 (2018): 70–84.

33. Yessica Ramos, "Brown Femme and Ace," in *Brown and Gray*, ed. jnramos, 2015.

34. Mark Carrigan, "There's More to Life Than Sex? Difference and Commonality within the Asexual Community," *Sexualities* 14, no. 4 (2011): 462–78.

35. Tucker, *(A)sexual*.

36. Lorca Jolene Sloan, "Ace of (BDSM) Clubs: Building Asexual Relationships through BDSM Practice," *Sexualities* 18, no. 5–6 (2015): 548–63.

37. KJ Cerankowski and M. Milks, eds., *Asexualities: Feminist and Queer Perspectives* (New York: Routledge, 2014).

38. Peter Cryle and Alison Moore, eds., *Frigidity: An Intellectual History* (New York: Palgrave Macmillan, 2012); Havelock Ellis, *Studies in the Psychology of Sex: Analysis of the Sexual Impulse, Love and Pain, and the Sexual Impulse in Women* (Philadelphia: Davis, 1912), 154; Donald W. Hastings, *Impotence and Frigidity* (Boston: Little, Brown, 1963); Richard von Krafft-Ebing, *Psychopathia Sexualis with Especial Reference to Contrary Sexual Instincts: A Clinical Forensic Study*, 12th ed., trans. Charles G. Chaddock (New York: Rebman, 1886/1922), 61–69; Harold Lief, "What's New in Sexual Research? Inhibited Sexual Desire," *Medical Aspects of Human Sexuality* 11 (1977): 94–95; American Psychiatric Association, *Diagnostic and Statistical Manual of Mental Disorders* (3rd edition, revised) (Washington, DC: APA, 1980); American Psychiatric Association, *Diagnostic and Statistical Manual of Mental Disorders*, 5th ed. (Arlington, VA: American Psychiatric Publishing, 2013). Also see Kim, "Asexualities and Disabilities in Constructing Sexual Normalcy."

39. Nancy F. Cott, "Passionlessness: An Interpretation of Victorian Sexual Ideology, 1790–1850," *Signs: Journal of Women in Culture and Society* 4, no. 2 (Winter 1978): 219–36.

40. Ianna Hawkins Owen, "On the Racialization of Asexuality," in *Asexualities: Feminist and Queer Perspectives*, ed. KJ Cerankowski and M. Milks (New York: Routledge, 2014), 125.

41. Kinsey, Pomeroy, and Martin, *Sexual Behavior in the Human Male*, 638, 647. For a more in-depth critique of Kinsey see Przybylo, "Producing Facts."

42. Kinsey, Pomeroy, and Martin, *Sexual Behavior in the Human Male*, 656; Alfred C. Kinsey, Wardell B. Pomeroy, Clyde E. Martin, and Paul H. Gebhard, *Sexual Behavior in the Human Female* (Philadelphia: W. B. Saunders, 1953), 472.

43. Michael Storms, "Theories of Sexual Orientation," *Journal of Personality and Social Psychology* 38, no. 5 (1980): 783–92; Michael Storms, "Sexual Orientation and Self-Perception," in *Advances in the Study of Communication and Affect, Vol. 5: Perception of Emotion in Self and Others*, ed. Patricia Pliner, Kirk R. Blankstein, and Irwin M. Spigel (New York: Plenum Press, 1979): 165–80.

44. Paula S. Nurius, "Mental Health Implications of Sexual Orientation," *The Journal of Sex Research* 19, no. 2 (1983): 119, 127, 126, 122.

45. William H. Masters, Virginia E. Johnson, and Robert C. Kolodny, *Masters and Johnson on Sex and Human Loving* (Boston: Little, Brown, 1986), 364, 365.

46. Masters, Johnson, and Kolodny, *Masters and Johnson on Sex and Human Loving*, 365.

47. Anthony Bogaert, "Asexuality: Prevalence and Associated Factors in a National Probability Sample," *Journal of Sex Research* 41, no. 3 (2004): 279–87; Anne M. Johnson, Jane Wadsworth, Kaye Wellings, Julia Field, and Sally Bradshaw, *Sexual Attitudes and Lifestyles* (London: Blackwell Scientific Publications, 1994), 185. Also see Anthony Bogaert, "Toward a Conceptual Understanding of Asexuality," *Review of General Psychology* 10, no. 3 (2006): 241–50; Anthony Bogaert, "Asexuality: Dysfunction or Variation?," in *Psychological Sexual Dysfunctions*, ed. Jayson M. Caroll and Marta K. Alena (New York: Nova Science Publishers, 2008): 9–13; Anthony Bogaert, *Understanding Asexuality* (Toronto: Rowman & Littlefield, 2012).

48. KJ Cerankowski, "Spectacular Asexuals"; Hawkins Owen, "On the Racialization of Asexuality"; Ela Przybylo and Danielle Cooper, "Asexual Resonances: Tracing a Queerly Asexual Archive," *GLQ: A Journal of Lesbian and Gay Studies* 20, no. 3 (2014): 297–318.

49. Bogaert, "Asexuality"; Bogaert, *Understanding Asexuality*.

50. Catherine Aicken, Catherine Mercer, and Jackie Cassell, "Who Reports Absence of Sexual Attraction in Britain? Evidence from National Probability Surveys," *Psychology & Sexuality* 4, no. 2 (2013): 121–35; Bogaert, "Asexuality"; Ellen Van Houdenhove, Luk Gijs, Guy T'Sjoen, and Paul Enzlin, "Asexuality: Few Facts, Many Questions," *Journal of Sex & Marital Therapy* 40 (2014): 175–92. Also see Dudley L. Poston Jr. and Amanda K. Baumle, "Patterns of Asexuality in the United States," *Demographic Research* 23 (2010): 509–30.

51. Both Aicken et al. and Bogaert look at the UK; Poston and Baumle look at the US. Aicken, Mercer, and Cassell, "Who Reports Absence of Sexual Attraction in Britain?"; Bogaert, "Asexuality"; Poston and Baumle, "Patterns of Asexuality in the United States." See Przybylo, "Crisis and Safety: The Asexual in Sexusociety," *Sexualities* 14, no. 4 (2011) 444–61 for further analysis, especially of Bogaert's results. Limited research exists on asexuality in non-Western contexts. Two exceptions include Milica Batričević and Andrej Cvetić, "Uncovering an A: Asexuality and Asexual Activism in Croatia and Serbia," in *Intersectionality and LGBT Activist Politics,* ed. Bojan Bilić and Sanja Kajinić (London: Palgrave Macmillan, 2016), 77–103 and Day Wong, "Asexuality in China's Sexual Revolution: Asexual Marriage as Coping Strategy," *Sexualities* 18, no. 1–2 (2015): 100–116.

52. Lori Brotto and Morag Yule, "Asexuality: Sexual Orientation, Paraphilia, Sexual Dysfunction, or None of the Above?" *Archives of Sexual Behavior* 46, no. 3 (2017): 619–27; Lori Brotto and Morag A. Yule, "Physiological and Subjective Sexual Arousal in Self-Identified Asexual Women," *Archives of Sexual Behavior* 40, no. 4 (2011): 699–712.

53. Morag Yule, Lori Brotto, and Boris Gorzalka, "A Validated Measure of No Sexual Attraction: The Asexuality Identification Scale," *Psychological Assessment* 27, no. 1 (2015): 148–60.

54. American Psychiatric Association, *Diagnostic and Statistical Manual of Mental Disorders,* 4th ed. (Washington, DC: American Psychiatric Press, 1994); American Psychiatric Association, *Diagnostic and Statistical Manual of Mental Disorders,* 5th ed.

55. Cerankowski and Milks, eds., *Asexualities.* For an early exploration of asexuality, see Myra T. Johnson, "Asexual and Autoerotic Women: Two Invisible Groups," in *The Sexually Oppressed,* ed. Harvey L. Gochros and Jean S. Gochros, 96–109 (New York: Association Press, 1977).

56. Przybylo and Cooper, "Asexual Resonances."

57. Przybylo and Cooper, "Asexual Resonances," 299.

58. Bogaert, *Understanding Asexuality,* 5.

59. Przybylo and Cooper, "Asexual Resonances."

60. Eunjung Kim, "How Much Sex Is Healthy? The Pleasures of Asexuality," in *Against Health: How Health Became the New Morality,* ed. Jonathan M. Metzl and Anna Kirkland (New York: New York University Press, 2010): 157–69; Eunjung Kim, "Asexuality in Disability Narratives," *Sexualities* 14, no. 4 (2011): 479–93.

61. Przybylo and Cooper, "Asexual Resonances."

62. Rich, "Compulsory Heterosexuality and Lesbian Existence." For discussions of the term "compulsory sexuality," see Emens, "Compulsory Sexuality" and Gupta, "Compulsory Sexuality." Similar to "compulsory sexuality," the term "sexual imperative" has also been in use including prior to the burgeoning of research on asexuality. See Wendy Hollway, "Gender Difference and the Production of Subjectivity (1984)," in *Changing the Subject: Psychology, Social Regulation and Subjectivity* (London: Routledge, 1998); Nicola Gavey, *Just Sex? The Cultural Scaffolding of Rape* (London: Routledge, 2005); Annie Potts, *The Science/Fiction of Sex: Feminist Deconstruction and the Vocabularies of Heterosex* (London: Routledge, 2002). Other terms in use include the following: A. K. Morrissey uses the term "sexualnormativity" in "Remedial Asexuality," 166–67; Przybylo uses the term

"sexusociety" in "Crisis and Safety"; and Kim draws on "sexual normalcy" in "Asexualities and Disabilities in Constructing Sexual Normalcy."

63. Emens, "Compulsory Sexuality"; Gupta, "Compulsory Sexuality"; Kim, "How Much Sex Is Healthy?" and "Asexuality in Disability Narratives."

64. Kim, "How Much Sex Is Healthy?"; Kim, "Asexuality in Disability Narratives"; Emily Lund and Bayley Johnson, "Asexuality and Disability: Strange but Compatible Bedfellows," *Sexuality and Disability* 33, no. 1 (2015): 123–32; Kristina Gupta, "Asexuality and Disability: Mutual Negation in *Adams v. Rice* and New Directions for Coalition Building.," in *Asexualities: Feminist and Queer Perspectives,* ed. KJ Cerankowski and M. Milks (New York: Routledge, 2014).

65. Douglas Crimp, *AIDS: Cultural Analysis/Cultural Activism* (Cambridge: MIT Press, 1988).

66. Lauren Berlant and Lee Edelman, *Sex, or the Unbearable* (Durham, NC: Duke University Press, 2012), 5.

67. Hawkins Owen, "On the Racialization of Asexuality."

68. Breanne Fahs, "Radical Refusals: On the Anarchist Politics of Women Choosing Asexuality," *Sexualities* 13, no. 4 (2010): 445–61.

69. Jennifer Nelson, *Women of Color and the Reproductive Rights Movement* (New York: New York University Press, 2003); see chapter 1.

70. Przybylo, "Crisis and Safety."

71. Also see Kristina Gupta and KJ Cerankowski, "Asexualities and Media," in *The Routledge Companion to Media, Sex, and Sexuality,* ed. Clarissa Smith, Feona Attwood, and Brian McNair (New York: Routledge, 2018), 19–26.

72. *House* (television series; Los Angeles: Fox Network, 2012).

73. Carter, *The Heart of Whiteness*; Hawkins Owen, "On the Racialization of Asexuality."

74. Carter, *The Heart of Whiteness,* 55.

75. Susie Scott and Matt Dawson, "Rethinking Asexuality: A Symbolic Interactionist Account," *Sexualities* 18, no. 1–2 (2015): 3–19.

76. Staci Newmahr, "Eroticism as Embodied Emotion: The Erotics of Renaissance Faire," *Symbolic Interaction* 37, no. 2 (2014): 211, 209.

77. Stella Sandford, "Sexually Ambiguous," *Angelaki* 11, no. 3 (2006): 43–59.

78. Plato, *Symposium,* trans C. J. Rowe (Warminster: Aris & Phillips, 1998).

79. Sigmund Freud, *Three Essays on the Theory of Sexuality,* trans. James Strachey (New York: Basic Books, 1905/1975).

80. Sandford, "Sexually Ambiguous," 48; Sigmund Freud, "Lecture 20" (1916–1917), in *Introductory Lectures on Psychoanalysis,* trans. James Strachey, Penguin Freud Library Volume 1 (London: Penguin, 1973), 344.

81. Sandford, "Sexually Ambiguous," 53.

82. Sigmund Freud, *Civilization and Its Discontents,* trans. James Strachey, 1930 (New York: Norton, 1961); Lynne Huffer, *Are the Lips a Grave? A Queer Feminist on the Ethics of Sex* (New York: Columbia University Press, 2013), 11.

83. Sandford, "Sexually Ambiguous."

84. Stella Sandford argues that "eros, in all its manifestations, is neither somatic nor psychical, neither 'sexual' nor 'non-sexual,' but both," "Sexually Ambiguous," 56.

85. Huffer, *Are the Lips a Grave?*

86. Huffer, *Are the Lips a Grave?,* 12.

87. Banu Subramaniam, *Ghost Stories for Darwin: The Science of Variation and the Politics of Diversity* (Champaign: University of Illinois Press, 2014); Foucault, *The History of Sexuality.*

88. Kristina Gupta, "'Screw Health': Representations of Sex as a Health-Promoting Activity in Medical and Popular Literature," *Journal of Medical Humanities* 32, no. 2 (2011): 127–40.

89. Lorde, "Uses of the Erotic."

90. Alexis De Veaux, *Warrior Poet: A Biography of Audre Lorde* (New York: W. W. Norton, 2004), 68, 129.

91. De Veaux, *Warrior Poet,* 200.

92. Audre Lorde and Adrienne Rich, "An Interview: Audre Lorde and Adrienne Rich" (1979), in *Sister Outsider,* 81–109 (Freedom, CA: The Crossing Press, 1984), 109.

93. Lorde, "Uses of the Erotic," 53.

94. Lorde, "Uses of the Erotic," 53, 59.

95. Sigmund Freud, "Female Sexuality," in *Standard Edition of the Complete Psychological Works V. 21 (1927–1931),* trans. James Strachey (London: Hogarth Press, 1961).

96. Lorde, "Uses of the Erotic," 56.

97. Lorde, "Uses of the Erotic," 59, 57.

98. Lorde, "Uses of the Erotic," 54.

99. Lorde, "Uses of the Erotic," 56.

100. Lorde, "Uses of the Erotic," 55.

101. Gayle Rubin, "Thinking Sex: Notes for a Radical Theory of the Politics of Sexuality," in *Pleasure and Danger: Exploring Female Sexuality,* ed. Carole S. Vance (London: Routledge and Kegan Paul, 1984), 275.

102. Lorde, "Uses of the Erotic," 57.

103. Lorde, "Uses of the Erotic," 57.

104. Awkward-Rich, "A Prude's Manifesto."

105. Peter Coviello, *Tomorrow's Parties: Sex and the Untimely in Nineteenth-Century America* (New York: New York University Press, 2013).

106. Coviello, *Tomorrow's Parties,* 19. Foucault, *The History of Sexuality.*

107. Kathryn Kent, *Making Girls into Women: American Women's Writing* (Durham, NC: Duke University Press, 2003).

108. Sharon Patricia Holland, *The Erotic Life of Racism* (Durham, NC: Duke University Press, 2012).

109. Tracy Bear, "Power in My Blood: Corporeal Sovereignty through the Praxis of an Indigenous Eroticanalysis" (PhD diss., University of Alberta, 2016), 114.

110. Rubin, "Thinking Sex," 275.

111. Qwo-Li Driskill, "Stolen from Our Bodies: First Nations Two-Spirits/Queers and the Journey to a Sovereign Erotic," *Studies in American Indian Literatures* 16, no. 2 (2004): 51.

112. Bear, "Power in My Blood."

113. Driskill, "Stolen from Our Bodies." Also see Mark Rifkin, "The Erotics of Sovereignty," in *Queer Indigenous Studies: Critical Interventions in Theory, Politics, and Literature,* ed. Qwo-Li Driskill, Chris Finley, Brian Joseph Gilley, and Scott Lauria Morgensen (Tucson: University of Arizona Press, 2011).

114. Mark Rifkin, *The Erotics of Sovereignty: Queer Native Writing in the Era of Self-Determination* (Minneapolis: University of Minnesota Press, 2012), 27.

115. Mireille Miller-Young, *A Taste for Brown Sugar: Black Women in Pornography* (Durham, NC: Duke University Press, 2014), 16.

116. Angela Willey, *Undoing Monogamy: The Politics of Science and the Possibilities of Biology* (Durham, NC: Duke University Press, 2016), 128–29.

117. L. H. Stallings, *Funk the Erotic: Transaesthetics and Black Sexual Cultures* (Champaign: University of Illinois Press, 2015), 3–4.

118. Stallings, *Funk the Erotic,* 1.

119. Przybylo and Cooper, "Asexual Resonances," 299.

120. Sedgwick, *Epistemology of the Closet,* 34–35.

121. Coviello, *Tomorrow's Parties,* 4.

122. Lorde, "Uses of the Erotic," 57.

123. Awkward-Rich, "A Prude's Manifesto."

124. Coviello, *Tomorrow's Parties*, 41.
125. For research and sources on chastity and celibacy politics in the first wave, see Benjamin Kahan, *Celibacies: American Modernism and Sexual Life* (Durham, NC: Duke University Press, 2013).
126. By using the term "nonsexualities," I am borrowing from Kristina Gupta's use of the term in "Picturing Space for Lesbian Nonsexualities: Rethinking Sex-Normative Commitments through *The Kids Are All Right* (2010)," *Journal of Lesbian Studies* 17, no. 1 (2013): 103–18.
127. Przybylo, "Producing Facts"; Scott and Dawson, "Rethinking Asexuality," 4.
128. Foucault, *The History of Sexuality*.
129. Esther Rothblum and Kathleen Brehony, eds., *Boston Marriages: Romantic but Asexual Relationships among Contemporary Lesbians* (Amherst: University of Massachusetts Press, 1993).
130. Kate Bolick, *Spinster: Making a Life of One's Own* (New York: Penguin, 2015); Michael Cobb, *Single: Arguments for the Uncoupled* (New York: New York University Press, 2012); Cryle and Moore, eds., *Frigidity*; Rachel Hills, *The Sex Myth* (New York: Simon & Schuster, 2015); Kahan, *Celibacies*.
131. Carla Freccero, *Queer/Early/Modern* (Durham, NC: Duke University Press, 2006), 4–5.
132. Berlant and Edelman, *Sex, or the Unbearable*, 7.
133. Maggie Nelson, *The Argonauts* (Minneapolis, MN: Graywolf Press, 2015).
134. Catherine Opie, *Self-Portrait/Nursing*, chromogenic print, 2004, https://artsandculture.google.com/asset/self-portrait-nursing/SgHoN6WNo_B8gw and *Self-Portrait/Cutting*, chromogenic print, 1993, https://artsandculture.google.com/asset/self-portrait-cutting/yQG2x2FpePzJXw; Vivek Shraya, *Trisha*, 2016, https://vivekshraya.com/visual/trisha/.
135. Noah Baumbach, dir., *Frances Ha* (New York: RT Features, 2012).

## NOTES TO CHAPTER 1

1. Maggie Jochild, "SISTERHOOD FEELS GOOD," *Meta Watershed*, 2010, http://maggiesmetawatershed.blogspot.ca/2010/12/sisterhood-feels-good.html.
2. Liza Cowan, "Response," *Meta Watershed*, 2010, http://maggiesmetawatershed.blogspot.ca/2010/12/sisterhood-feels-good.html. The note is signed as "Liza," but I believe it was left by Liza Cowan.
3. Lorde, "Uses of the Erotic."
4. This comment is used with permission from the student who wished to remain unnamed. This assignment was modeled on one discussed by Bear in her dissertation, "Power in My Blood."
5. Lorde, "Uses of the Erotic," 55.
6. Lorde, "Uses of the Erotic," 59.
7. Lorde, "Uses of the Erotic," 59.
8. I use the terms separately when the primary sources refer to one over the other, and otherwise I indicate "political celibacy/asexuality" so as to emphasize the boundedness of these terms in the historical moment.
9. Toni Cade Bambara, "On the Issue of Roles" (1969/1970), in *The Black Woman: An Anthology*, ed. Toni Cade Bambara (New York: New American Library, 1970), 101.
10. Nelson, *Women of Color*, 118–19.
11. Interestingly, some suggest that Andy Warhol was himself asexual. See Ti-Grace Atkinson in interview with Breanne Fahs, "Ti-Grace Atkinson and the Legacy of Radical Feminism," *Feminist Studies* 37, no. 3 (2011): 576. Also see Breanne Fahs, *Valerie Solanas* (New York: The Feminist Press, 2014).

12. Finn Enke, "Collective Memory and Transfeminist 1970s: Toward a Less Plausible History," *TSQ: Transgender Studies Quarterly* 5, no. 1 (2018): 22–23; Cristan Williams, "Radical Inclusion: Recounting the Trans Inclusive History of Radical Feminism" *TSQ: Transgender Studies Quarterly* 3, no. 1–2 (2016): 255–56.

13. Ti-Grace Atkinson helped initiate the statement "Forbidden Discourse: The Silencing of Feminist Criticism of 'Gender,'" (2013) which neither Dana Densmore or Roxanne Dunbar-Ortiz agreed to sign. See it online at *Fire in My Belly: A Radical Feminist Blog*, https://feministuk.wordpress.com/2013/08/19/forbidden-discourse-the-silencing-of-feminist-criticism-of-gender/. Also see Breanne Fahs, *Firebrand Feminism: The Radical Lives of Ti-Grace Atkinson, Kathie Sarachild, Roxanne Dunbar-Ortiz, and Dana Densmore* (Washington, DC: University of Washington Press, 2018), 160.

14. The Young Lords Party worked with trans women, and Sylvia Rivera was involved in their lesbian and gay caucus. Leslie Feinberg, "Street Transvestite Action Revolutionaries," *Workers World*, 2006, http://www.workers.org/2006/us/lavender-red-73/.

15. Fahs, "Radical Refusals."

16. Fahs, "Radical Refusals," 446–47.

17. Based on conversations I had with Fahs, in which she discussed the negative pushback she received for publishing "Radical Refusals."

18. Kim, "Asexualities and Disabilities in Constructing Sexual Normalcy," 274.

19. KJ Cerankowski and M. Milks, "New Orientations: Asexuality and Its Implications for Theory and Practice," *Feminist Studies* 36, no. 3 (2010): 656.

20. Victoria Hesford, "Feminism and Its Ghosts: The Spectre of the Feminist-as-Lesbian," *Feminist Theory* 6, no. 3 (2005): 238, 239.

21. Jane Gerhard, *Desiring Revolution: Second Wave Feminism and the Rewriting of American Sexual Thought, 1920 to 1982* (New York: Columbia University Press, 2001), 2.

22. William H. Masters and Virginia E. Johnson, *Human Sexual Response* (New York: Bantam Books, 1966). Also see Janice M. Irvine, *Disorders of Desire: Sexuality and Gender in Modern American Sexology* (Philadelphia: Temple University Press, 1990/2005), 60–66.

23. Gavey, *Just Sex?*, 108.

24. Steven Seidman, *Romantic Longings: Love in America, 1830–1980* (New York: Routledge, 1991), 122. Helen Gurley Brown, *Sex and the Single Girl: The Unmarried Woman's Guide to Men* (New York: Pocket Books, 1962); John D'Emilio and Estelle B. Freedman, *Intimate Matters: A History of Sexuality in America* (New York: Harper and Row, 1988); Lisa Maria Hogeland, "Sexuality in the Consciousness-Raising Novel of the 1970s," *Journal of the History of Sexuality* 5, no. 4 (1995): 601–32.

25. Atkinson, in interview with Fahs, "Ti-Grace Atkinson and the Legacy of Radical Feminism," 573; Gavey, *Just Sex?*, 108.

26. Roxanne Dunbar-Ortiz, "'Sexual Liberation': More of the Same Thing," *No More Fun and Games* 3 (1969): 49–50.

27. Hawkins Owen, "On the Racialization of Asexuality."

28. Daniel Patrick Moynihan, *The Negro Family: The Case for National Action* (Washington, DC: GPO, 1965).

29. Patricia Hill Collins, *Black Feminist Thought: Knowledge, Consciousness, and the Politics of Empowerment* (New York: Routledge, 1990), 71.

30. Hawkins Owen, "On the Racialization of Asexuality."

31. Collins, *Black Feminist Thought*.

32. Dorothy E. Roberts, *Killing the Black Body: Race, Reproduction, and the Meaning of Liberty* (New York: Pantheon Books, 1997).

33. Nelly Oudshoorn, *Beyond the Natural Body: An Archaeology of Sex Hormones* (New York: Routledge, 1994), 112–37.

34. Sally Torpy, "Native American Woman and Coerced Sterilization: On the Trail of Tears in the 1970s," *American Indian Culture and Research Journal* 24, no. 2 (2000): 1–22.

35. Toni Cade Bambara, "The Pill: Genocide or Liberation?," in *The Black Woman: An Anthology*, ed. Toni Cade Bambara (New York: New American Library, 1970), 163; Margo Natalie Crawford, "Must Revolution Be a Family Affair? Revisiting *The Black Woman*," in *Want to Start a Revolution?: Radical Women in the Black Freedom Struggle*, ed. Dayo F. Gore, Jeanne Theoharis, and Komozi Woodard (New York: New York University Press, 2009), 196. Also see Young Lords Party, *Palante* 2, no. 10 (1970): 5.

36. Winifred Breines, *The Trouble Between Us: An Uneasy History of White and Black Women in the Feminist Movement* (Oxford: Oxford University Press, 2006), 40.

37. Kimberly Springer, *Living for the Revolution: Black Feminist Organizations, 1968–1980* (Durham, NC: Duke University Press, 2005).

38. Springer, *Living for the Revolution*, 29.

39. Gore, Theoharis, and Woodard, eds. *Want to Start a Revolution?*

40. Sherie M. Randolph, *Florynce "Flo" Kennedy: The Life of a Black Feminist Radical* (Chapel Hill: University of North Carolina Press, 2015).

41. Frances Beale, "Double Jeopardy: To Be Black and Female," in *The Black Woman: An Anthology*, ed. Toni Cade Bambara (New York: New American Library, 1970), 90–100; Third World Women's Alliance, "Goals and Objectives," *Triple Jeopardy* (September–October 1971): 8; Springer, *Living for the Revolution*, 114 and 33.

42. Toni Cade Bambara, preface in *The Black Woman: An Anthology*, ed. Toni Cade Bambara (New York: New American Library, 1970), 7–12.

43. Combahee River Collective, "A Black Feminist Statement," in *All the Women Are White, All the Blacks Are Men, But Some of Us Are Brave: Black Women's Studies*, ed. Gloria T. Hull, Patricia Bell Scott, and Barbara Smith (Old Westbury, NY: The Feminist Press, 1982), 13.

44. Ianna Hawkins Owen, "Asexuality, Incarceration, and Black Power(lessness)," presented November 18, 2017, at the National Women's Studies Association annual conference.

45. Robin Kelley, *Freedom Dreams: The Black Radical Imagination* (Boston: Beacon Press, 2002). Also see Gore, Theoharis, Woodard, *Want to Start a Revolution?*, 6.

46. Kent, *Making Girls into Women*, 21–22.

47. Pauline Hopkins, "Higher Education of Colored Women in White Schools and Colleges (1902)," in *Daughter of the Revolution*, ed. Ira Dworkin (New Brunswick, NJ: Rutgers University Press, 2007), 198. See Kahan, *Celibacies*, 94.

48. Hawkins Owen, "Asexuality, Incarceration, and Black Power(lessness)." Hawkins Owen notes that even while Huggins reported wanting to feel connection, "sex was not at the top of her list."

49. Jean Carey Bond and Patricia Peery, "Is the Black Male Castrated?," in *The Black Woman: An Anthology*, ed. Toni Cade Bambara (New York: New American Library, 1970), 115.

50. Crawford, "Must Revolution Be a Family Affair?," 192.

51. Gwen Patton, "Black People and the Victorian Ethos," in *The Black Woman: An Anthology*, ed. Toni Cade Bambara (New York: New American Library, 1970), 147.

52. More recently, during a talk at The New School, bell hooks also mentioned celibacy, directly indicating that she had been celibate for fifteen years; "to [her], celibacy does not mean [she's] not sexual." bell hooks, "Are you Still A Slave? Liberating the Black Female Body" (New York: The New School, 2014).

53. Kahan, *Celibacies*, 81–98.

54. Kahan, *Celibacies*, 91.

55. Kahan, *Celibacies*, 86.

56. Kahan, *Celibacies*, 90.

57. Bambara, "On the Issue of Roles," 101–10.

58. Brittney Cooper, *Beyond Respectability: The Intellectual Thought of Race Women* (Urbana: University of Illinois Press, 2017), 130.

59. Farah Jasmine Griffin, "Conflict and Chorus: Reconsidering Toni Cade's *The Black Woman: An Anthology*," in *Is It Nation Time?: Contemporary Essays on Black Power and Black Nationalism,* ed. Eddie S. Glaude (Chicago: The University of Chicago Press, 2002); Cooper, *Beyond Respectability.*

60. Bambara, "On the Issue of Roles."

61. Bambara, "On the Issue of Roles," 101.

62. Bambara, "On the Issue of Roles," 105.

63. Patton, "Black People and the Victorian Ethos," 145.

64. Bambara, "On the Issue of Roles," 106.

65. Bambara, "On the Issue of Roles," 109.

66. Bambara, "On the Issue of Roles," 101.

67. Bambara, "On the Issue of Roles," 109.

68. Audre Lorde, "Sexism: An American Disease in Blackface" (1979), in *Sister Outsider* (Freedom, CA: The Crossing Press, 1984), 64–65; Audre Lorde, "Scratching the Surface: Some Notes on Barriers to Women and Loving" (1978), in *Sister Outsider* (Freedom, CA: The Crossing Press, 1984), 46.

69. Bob Bennett, "(Title)," in *Black Fire: An Anthology of Afro-American Writing,* ed. LeRoi Jones and Larry Neal (New York: William Morrow, 1968), 423. See Crawford, "Must Revolution Be a Family Affair?," 200–201.

70. Crawford, "Must Revolution Be a Family Affair?," 200.

71. Crawford, "Must Revolution Be a Family Affair?," 200.

72. Bennett, "(Title)," 423; Brake, *Minimizing Marriage.*

73. Johanna Fernández, "Denise Oliver and the Young Lords Party: Stretching the Political Boundaries of Struggle," in *Want to Start a Revolution?: Radical Women in the Black Freedom Struggle,* ed. Dayo F. Gore, Jeanne Theoharis, and Komozi Woodard (New York: New York University Press, 2009), 271–93.

74. Fernández, "Denise Oliver and the Young Lords Party," 281; Darrel Enck-Wanzer, ed. *The Young Lords: A Reader* (New York: New York University Press, 2010).

75. Young Lords Party, "Thirteen Point Program and Platform / Programa de 13 Puntos y Plataforma," *Palante* 2, no. 2 (1970): 18–19. Available online at https://www.marxists.org/history/erol/ncm-1/palante/.

76. Young Lords Party, "Young Lords Party Position Paper on Women," *Palante* 2, no. 12 (1970): 12.

77. Denise Oliver, "We Were Young Lords, Not Young Ladies," *Daily Kos* (August 22, 2009): https://www.dailykos.com/stories/2009/8/22/770157/—.

78. Iris Morales, "¡Palante, Siempre Palante! The Young Lords," in *The Puerto Rican Movement: Voices from the Diaspora,* ed. Andrés Torres and José E. Velázquez (Philadelphia: Temple University Press, 1998), 219.

79. Nelson, *Women of Color,* 118–19.

80. Young Lords Party, *Palante* 2, no. 15 (1970): 22; Fernández, "Denise Oliver and the Young Lords Party," 288.

81. Young Lords Party, "Young Lords Party Position Paper on Women," 14.

82. The sex strike issued by the women of the YLP was represented in the fictional Lysistrata-type rebellion in Spike Lee's satire film *Chi-Raq* (2015), where the women chant "No Peace, No Pussy" and band together to refuse men sex as a form of opposition to violence in Chicago's Southside.

83. Collins, *Black Feminist Thought,* 166.

84. Valerie Solanas, "SCUM (Society for Cutting Up Men) Manifesto" (1967), in *Radical Feminism: A Documentary Reader,* ed. Barbara Crow (New York: New York University Press, 2000), 201–22.

85. Fahs, *Valerie Solanas,* 47.

86. Lorde, "Uses of the Erotic," 58.
87. Fahs, *Firebrand Feminism*, 141.
88. The language of the "killjoy" is from Sara Ahmed's seminal piece, "Killing Joy: Feminism and the History of Happiness," *Signs: Journal of Women in Culture and Society* 35, no. 3 (2010): 571–94.
89. Solanas, "SCUM," 211.
90. Solanas, "SCUM," 213.
91. Solanas, "SCUM," 217.
92. Solanas, "SCUM," 213.
93. Solanas, "SCUM," 220.
94. Solanas, "SCUM," 217
95. Fahs, *Valerie Solanas*.
96. Betty Friedan, *It Changed My Life: Writings on the Women's Movement* (New York: Random House, 1976), 108. Fahs, *Valerie Solanas*, 163, 183–84.
97. Robin Morgan, ed., *Sisterhood Is Powerful: An Anthology of Writings from the Women's Liberation Movement* (New York: Random House, 1970); Alice Echols, *Daring to Be Bad: Radical Feminism in America, 1967–1975* (Minneapolis: University of Minnesota Press, 1989), 105; Fahs, *Valerie Solanas*, 176–88; Randolph, *Florynce "Flo" Kennedy*, 143–51.
98. Interview with Charlotte Bunch in Echols, *Daring to Be Bad*, 104.
99. Interview with Charlotte Bunch in Echols, *Daring to Be Bad*, 105.
100. Anne Koedt, "The Myth of the Vaginal Orgasm," in *Notes from the Second Year: Women's Liberation* (New York: New York Radical Feminists, 1968/1970), 37–41; Echols, *Daring to Be Bad*, 106–11.
101. Echols, *Daring to Be Bad*, 111.
102. Cited in Echols, *Daring to Be Bad*, 111.
103. Randolph, *Florynce "Flo" Kennedy*, esp. 122–26.
104. Lorde, "Uses of the Erotic," 55.
105. Lorde, "Uses of the Erotic," 56, 55.
106. Sherie M. Randolph, "'Women's Liberation or . . . Black Liberation, You're Fighting the Same Enemies': Florynce Kennedy, Black Power, and Feminism," in *Want to Start a Revolution?: Radical Women in the Black Freedom Struggle*, ed. Dayo F. Gore, Jeanne Theoharis, and Komozi Woodard (New York: New York University Press, 2009), 241.
107. Randolph, "'Women's Liberation or . . . Black Liberation, You're Fighting the Same Enemies," 242.
108. Randolph, *Florynce "Flo" Kennedy*, 163–64.
109. Randolph, *Florynce "Flo" Kennedy*, 165–66.
110. Koedt, "The Myth of the Vaginal Orgasm."
111. The Feminists, "The Feminists: A Political Organization to Annihilate Sex Roles," in *Notes from the Second Year: Women's Liberation*, ed. Shulamith Firestone and Anne Koedt (New York: New York Radical Feminists, 1970), 116–17. See also Echols, *Daring to Be Bad*, 176; Ti-Grace Atkinson, "Radical Feminism and Love," in *Amazon Odyssey: The First Collection of Writings by the Political Pioneer of the Women's Movement* (New York: Link Books, 1969/1974), 44; The Feminists, "Dangers in the Pro-Women Line" (New York: The Feminists, mimeograph, n.d.), 5.
112. The Feminists, "The Feminists: A Political Organization to Annihilate Sex Roles," 117.
113. Ti-Grace Atkinson, "The Institution of Sexual Intercourse," *Notes from the Second Year: Women's Liberation* (New York: New York Radical Feminists, 1970), 44–45.
114. Ti-Grace Atkinson, "Lesbianism and Feminism: Justice for Women as 'Unnatural,'" in *Amazon Odyssey: The First Collection of Writings by the Political Pioneer of the Women's Movement* (New York: Link Books, 1970/1974), 85.
115. Echols, *Daring to Be Bad*, 173.

116. Simone de Beauvoir, *The Second Sex* (New York: Vintage Books, 1949/2012).

117. Susan Rennie and Kirsten Grimstad, *The New Woman's Survival Catalogue* (New York: Coward, McCann and Geoghegan, 1973), 209.

118. Interview with Pam Kearon in Echols, *Daring to Be Bad*, 182.

119. Fahs, "Radical Refusals," 448.

120. Echols, *Daring to Be Bad*, 162.

121. Roxanne Dunbar-Ortiz, "Female Liberation as the Basis for Social Revolution," *No More Fun and Games* 2 (1969): 111.

122. Dana Densmore, "Sexuality," *No More Fun and Games* 1 (1968/1970): not paginated.

123. Indra Allen, "Why I Am Celibate (Interview with Indra Allen by Dana Densmore)," *No More Fun and Games* 6 (1972/1973): 39–46; Dana Densmore, "On Celibacy," *No More Fun and Games* 1 (1968/1970): not paginated; Dana Densmore, "Independence from the Sexual Revolution," *Notes from the Third Year: Women's Liberation* (New York: New York Radical Feminists, 1971), 56–61; Roxanne Dunbar-Ortiz, "Asexuality," *No More Fun and Games* 1 (1968/1970): not paginated; Roxanne Dunbar-Ortiz, "Sexual Liberation"; Ellen O'Donnell, "Thoughts on Celibacy," *No More Fun and Games* 1 (1968/1970): not paginated.

124. Densmore, "On Celibacy," not paginated.

125. Densmore, "Independence from the Sexual Revolution," 58.

126. Densmore, "Independence from the Sexual Revolution," 58.

127. Densmore, "Independence from the Sexual Revolution," 59.

128. Densmore, "Independence from the Sexual Revolution," 59.

129. Rubin, "Thinking Sex," 278.

130. Also see Barbara Lipschutz, "Nobody Needs to Get Fucked," *Lesbian Voices* 1, no. 4 (1975): 57. Lipschutz reimagines what can count as sex and intimacy: "An aspect of sexual liberation is freeing the libido from the tyranny of orgasm-seeking. Sometimes hugging is nicer. . . . Holding hands is love-making. Touching lips is love-making. Rubbing breasts is love-making. Locking souls with women by looking deep in their eyes is love-making."

131. Densmore, "On Celibacy," not paginated.

132. Densmore, "Independence from the Sexual Revolution," 56.

133. Densmore, "Independence from the Sexual Revolution," 56.

134. Rita Mae Brown, *A Plain Brown Rapper* (Oakland, CA: Diana Press, 1976), 50.

135. Anne M. Valk, "Living a Feminist Lifestyle: The Intersection of Theory and Action in a Lesbian Feminist Collective," *Feminist Studies* 28, no. 2 (2002): 303–32; Rita Mae Brown, *Rubyfruit Jungle* (New York: Bantam Books, 1973).

136. Radicalesbians, "The Woman Identified Woman," in *Notes from the Third Year: Women's Liberation* (New York: New York Radical Feminists, 1970/1971), 81–84; Echols, *Daring to Be Bad*, 214–15.

137. Echols, *Daring to Be Bad*, 216.

138. Ginny Berson, "The Furies," in *Lesbianism and the Women's Movement*, ed. The Furies, Nancy Myron, and Charlotte Bunch (Baltimore: Diana Press, 1975), 18.

139. Echols, *Daring to Be Bad*, 217.

140. Ginny Z. Berson, "The Furies: Goddesses of Vengeance," *Serials Review* 16, no. 4 (1990): 79–87.

141. Berson, "The Furies: Goddesses of Vengeance."

142. Berson, "The Furies: Goddesses of Vengeance."

143. Sue Katz, "Smash Phallic Imperialism" (sometimes printed as "The Sensuous Woman"), in *Out of the Closets: Voices of Gay Liberation*, ed. Karla Jay and Allen Young (New York: New York University Press, 1971/1992), 259–62.

144. Sue Negrin, "A Weekend in Lesbian Nation," *It Ain't Me, Babe* 2, no. 1 (1971): 11; Echols, *Daring to Be Bad*, 346n62.

145. Women's Commune, "Mind Bogglers," *Off Our Backs* 1, no. 9/10 (1970): 13. Also, Carol Anne Douglas writes sympathetically of celibacy in several pieces in *Off Our Backs:* see Carol Anne Douglas, "Interview: Dana Densmore: Self-Defense and Feminism," *Off Our Backs* 5, no. 1 (1975): 8–9, 19 and Carol Anne Douglas and Alice Henry, "Towards a Politics of Sexuality," *Off Our Backs* 12, no. 6 (1982): 2–4, 20–21.

146. Lorde, "Uses of the Erotic," 55.

## NOTES TO CHAPTER 2

1. Brigitte Lewis, "The Era of Lesbian Bed Death Is Over, Long Live Lesbian Fuck Eye," *Archer Magazine,* September 9, 2015, http://archermagazine.com.au/2015/09/the-era-of-lesbian-bed-death-is-over-long-live-lesbian-fuck-eye/.

2. Lewis, "The Era of Lesbian Bed Death Is Over," n. p.

3. Philip Blumstein and Pepper Schwartz, *American Couples: Money, Work, Sex* (New York: William Morrow, 1983).

4. Berlant and Edelman, *Sex, or the Unbearable,* 8.

5. Berlant and Edelman, *Sex, or the Unbearable,* 3.

6. Lewis, "The Era of Lesbian Bed Death Is Over," n. p.

7. Blumstein and Schwartz, *American Couples,* 18.

8. Blumstein and Schwartz, *American Couples,* 197.

9. Blumstein and Schwartz, *American Couples,* 197, 214.

10. Jo-Ann Krestan and Claudia Bepko, "The Problem of Fusion in the Lesbian Relationship," *Family Process* 19, no. 3 (1980): 277–89. Also see Margaret Nichols, "The Treatment of Inhibited Sexual Desire (ISD) in Lesbian Couples," *Women & Therapy* 1, no. 4 (1982): 49–66.

11. Gupta, "Picturing Space for Lesbian Nonsexualities," 105; Suzanne Iasenza, "Lesbian Sexuality Post-Stonewall to Post-Modernism: Putting the 'Lesbian Bed Death' Concept to Bed," *Journal of Sex Education and Therapy* 25, no. 1 (2000): 60.

12. Iasenza, "Lesbian Sexuality Post-Stonewall to Post-Modernism," 59. For other critiques of lesbian bed death, see Marilyn Frye, "Lesbian 'Sex,'" in *Willful Virgin: Essays in Feminism, 1976–1992* (Freedom, CA: Crossing Press, 1992); Gupta, "Picturing Space for Lesbian Nonsexualities"; Michele O'Mara, "The Correlation of Sexual Frequency and Relationship Satisfaction Among Lesbians" (PhD diss., American Academy of Clinical Sexologists, Florida, 2012).

13. Gupta, "Picturing Space for Lesbian Nonsexualities," 105.

14. Jacqueline Cohen and Sandra Byers, "Beyond Lesbian Bed Death: Enhancing Our Understanding of the Sexuality of Sexual-Minority Women in Relationships," *Journal of Sex Research* 51, no. 8 (2014): 893–903.

15. Jade McGleughlin in an interview with O'Mara. O'Mara, "The Correlation of Sexual Frequency and Relationship Satisfaction Among Lesbians," 82.

16. Jade McGleughlin in an interview with O'Mara. O'Mara, "The Correlation of Sexual Frequency and Relationship Satisfaction Among Lesbians," 82–83.

17. Studies that contradict Schwartz and Blumstein's findings include Lauren Bressler and Abraham Lavender, "Sexual Fulfillment of Heterosexual, Bisexual, and Homosexual Women," in *Historical, Literary, and Erotic Aspects of Lesbianism,* ed. Monika Kehoe (New York: Haworth Press, 1986); Cohen and Byers, "Beyond Lesbian Bed Death"; Emily Coleman, Peter Hoon, and Emily Hoon, "Arousability and Sexual Satisfaction in Lesbian and Heterosexual Women," *Journal of Sex Research* 19, no. 1 (1983): 58–73; Jack Hedblom, "Dimensions of Lesbian Sexual Experience," *Archives of Sexual Behavior* 2, no. 4 (1973): 329–41; William Masters and Virginia Johnson, *Homosexuality in Perspective* (Boston: Little, Brown, 1979). See Iasenza, "Lesbian Sexuality Post-Stonewall to Post-Modernism."

18. Iasenza, "Lesbian Sexuality Post-Stonewall to Post-Modernism," 61–62. See also Blumstein and Schwartz, *American Couples*, 197.
19. Cohen and Byers, "Beyond Lesbian Bed Death."
20. Iasenza, "Lesbian Sexuality Post-Stonewall to Post-Modernism," 62.
21. Iasenza, "Lesbian Sexuality Post-Stonewall to Post-Modernism," 62.
22. Gupta, "Picturing Space for Lesbian Nonsexualities"; Frye, "Lesbian 'Sex'"; O'Mara, "The Correlation of Sexual Frequency and Relationship Satisfaction Among Lesbians."
23. For an elaboration of sexunormativity see Przybylo, "Crisis and Safety," 444–61.
24. Lewis, "The Era of Lesbian Bed Death Is Over." See also Gupta, "Picturing Space for Lesbian Nonsexualities."
25. Blumstein and Schwartz, *American Couples*, 198.
26. Alison Bechdel, *The Essential Dykes to Watch Out For* (Boston, New York: Houghton Mifflin Harcourt, 2008); Jenji Kohan, prod., *Orange Is the New Black* (television series; Santa Monica: Lionsgate Television, 2013); Peter Paige et al., prod., *The Fosters* (television series; Burbank: ABC Family, 2013); Lisa Cholodenko, dir., *The Kids Are All Right* (Los Angeles: Gilbert Films, 2010).
27. Rebecca Beirne, *Lesbians in Television and Text After the Millennium* (London: Palgrave Macmillan, 2008).
28. Cobb, *Single*. Also see Meg Barker and Darren Langdridge, eds., *Understanding Non-Monogamies* (London: Routledge, 2010).
29. Caleb Luna, "Romantic Love Is Killing Us: Who Takes Care of Us When We Are Single?," *The Body Is Not An Apology*, 2016, https://thebodyisnotanapology.com/magazine/romantic-love-is-killing-us/.
30. Lauren Berlant, *Cruel Optimism* (Durham, NC: Duke University Press, 2011).
31. Russell Shuttleworth, "Bridging Theory and Experience: A Critical-Interpretive Ethnography of Sexuality and Disability," in *Sex and Disability*, ed. Robert McRuer and Anna Mollow (Durham, NC: Duke University Press, 2012), 176.
32. Leo Bersani, "Is the Rectum a Grave?" *October* 43 (1987): 197–222; Michael Warner, *The Trouble with Normal: Sex, Politics, and the Ethics of Queer Life* (Cambridge, MA: Harvard University Press, 2000).
33. Thea Cacchioni, "Heterosexuality and 'the Labour of Love': A Contribution to Recent Debates on Female Sexual Dysfunction," *Sexualities* 10, no. 3 (2007): 299–320; Gupta, "Screw Health." Also see Kristina Gupta and Thea Cacchioni, "Sexual Improvement as if Your Health Depends on It: An Analysis of Contemporary Sex Manuals," *Feminism & Psychology* 23, no. 4 (2013): 442–58; Kim, "How Much Sex Is Healthy?"; Judy Segal, "The Sexualization of the Medical," *Journal of Sex Research* 49, no. 4 (2012): 369–78.
34. Cynthia Barounis, "Compulsory Sexuality and Asexual/Crip Resistance in John Cameron Mitchell's *Shortbus*," in *Asexualities: Feminist and Queer Perspectives*, ed. KJ Cerankowski and M. Milks (New York: Routledge, 2014).
35. Gupta, "Picturing Space for Lesbian Nonsexualities."
36. Jack Halberstam, "The Kids Aren't Alright!," *Bully Bloggers*, July 15, 2010, http://bullybloggers.wordpress.com/2010/07/15/the-kids-arent-alright/.
37. Gupta, "Picturing Space for Lesbian Nonsexualities."
38. Warner, *The Trouble with Normal*, 89.
39. Barounis, "Compulsory Sexuality and Asexual/Crip Resistance."
40. Barounis, "Compulsory Sexuality and Asexual/Crip Resistance," 175.
41. Terry Castle, *The Apparitional Lesbian: Female Homosexuality and Modern Culture* (New York: Columbia University Press, 1993), 2, 10.
42. Lorde, "Uses of the Erotic."
43. Barbara Smith, "Toward a Black Feminist Criticism," (1977) *Women's Studies International Quarterly* 2, no. 2 (1979): 183–94.
44. Smith, "Toward a Black Feminist Criticism"; Rich, "Compulsory Heterosexuality and Lesbian Existence"; Radicalesbians, "The Woman Identified Woman."

45. Lillian Faderman, *Surpassing the Love of Men: Romantic Friendship and Love between Women from the Renaissance to the Present* (New York: William Morrow, 1981); Martha Vicinus, *Intimate Friends: Women Who Loved Women, 1778–1928* (Chicago: University of Chicago Press, 2004); Omise'eke Natasha Tinsley, *Thiefing Sugar: Eroticism between Women in Caribbean Literature* (Durham, NC: Duke University Press, 2010).

46. Vicinus, *Intimate Friends,* xx.

47. Faderman, *Surpassing the Love of Men*; Rothblum and Brehony, *Boston Marriages.*

48. Faderman, *Surpassing the Love of Men,* 17–18. Similarly, Vicinus sees intimate friendship as "an emotional, *erotically* charged relationship between two women": Vicinus, *Intimate Friends,* xxiv, emphasis added.

49. Tinsley, *Thiefing Sugar,* 20.

50. Leslie Feinberg, *Stone Butch Blues* (Ithaca, NY: Firebrand Books, 1993).

51. Harmony Hammond, *Lesbian Art in America: A Contemporary History* (New York: Rizzoli, 2000).

52. Nancy Fraser, "Rethinking the Public Sphere: A Contribution to the Critique of Actually Existing Democracy," *Social Text* 25, no. 26 (1990): 56–80; Michael Warner, *Publics and Counterpublics* (Cambridge, MA: MIT Press, 2002).

53. Dana Seitler, "Making Sexuality Sensible: Tammy Rae Carland's and Catherine Opie's Queer Aesthetic Forms," in *Feeling Photography,* ed. Elspeth H. Brown and Thy Phu (Durham, NC: Duke University Press, 2014). See also Kenneth Silver, "Master Bedrooms, Master Narratives: Home, Homosexuality, and Post-War Art," in *Not at Home: The Suppression of Domesticity in Modern Art and Architecture,* ed. Christopher Reed (London: Thames and Hudson, 1996), 209.

54. For the entire series, visit Tammy Rae Carland's website: http://www.tammyraecarland.com/lesbianbeds.htm.

55. "Tammy Rae Carland: Lesbian Beds," *A Simple, Frugal Heart Blog,* 2011, http://thistlebirdhex.tumblr.com/post/13747149601/tammy-rae-carland-lesbian-beds-the-series-was.

56. Silver, "Master Bedrooms, Master Narratives," 215. For a discussion of Rauschenberg's relationship with Jasper Johns, see Jonathan Katz, "The Art of Code," in *Significant Others,* ed. Whotney Chadwick and Isabelle de Courtivron (New York: Thames and Hudson, 1993), available online at http://www.queer-arts.org/archive/show4/forum/katz/katz_set.html.

57. Silver, "Master Bedrooms, Master Narratives," 215.

58. "'It's Not a Viewing Platform, It's an Experience': Tracey Emin Prepares to Put Bed on View at Tate Britain," *Culture24,* March 20, 2015, http://www.culture24.org.uk/art/art522146-not-a-viewing-platform-an-experience-tracey-emin-prepares-to-put-bed-on-view-at-tate-britain.

59. "It's Not a Viewing Platform, It's an Experience."

60. "Tammy Rae Carland: Lesbian Beds."

61. For Kyle Lasky's entire series, visit http://www.kylelasky.com/lesbian-bedrooms-ii.

62. "A Record of 'Lesbian Bedrooms': An Interview with Photographer Kyle Lasky—NMP," *No More Potlucks* 22 (2012), http://nomorepotlucks.org/site/record-lesbian-bedrooms/.

63. "A Record of 'Lesbian Bedrooms.'"

64. Lee Wallace, *Lesbianism, Cinema, Space: The Sexual Life of Apartments* (New York: Routledge, 2009), 11.

65. Wallace, *Lesbianism, Cinema, Space,* 130.

66. Lauren Berlant and Michael Warner, "Sex in Public," *Critical Inquiry* 24, no. 2 (1998): 547–66. For critiques of the political prioritizing of public sex, see Wallace, *Lesbianism, Cinema, Space* and Christopher Castiglia, "Sex Panics, Sex Publics, Sex Memories," *Boundary 2* 27, no. 2 (2000): 149–75.

67. Wallace, *Lesbianism, Cinema, Space,* 133.

68. Seitler, "Making Sexuality Sensible," 47.

69. Barounis, "Compulsory Sexuality and Asexual/Crip Resistance"; Halberstam, "The Kids Aren't Alright!"

70. Erica Chu, "Radical Identity Politics: Asexuality and Contemporary Articulations of Identity," in *Asexualities: Feminist and Queer Perspectives*, ed. KJ Cerankowski and M. Milks (New York: Routledge, 2014), 83.

71. Barounis, "Compulsory Sexuality and Asexual/Crip Resistance"; Gupta, "Asexuality and Disability"; Kim, "Asexualities and Disabilities in Constructing Sexual Normalcy"; Lund and Johnson, "Asexuality and Disability."

72. Berlant and Edelman, *Sex, or the Unbearable*, 3.

73. Berlant and Edelman, *Sex, or the Unbearable*, 4.

74. Lisa Duggan, *The Twilight of Equality* (Boston, Beacon Press, 2003), 50; Heather Love, "Compulsory Happiness and Queer Existence," *New Formations* 63 (2007): 52–64.

75. Love, "Compulsory Happiness and Queer Existence," 54.

76. Jasbir Puar, *Terrorist Assemblages: Homonationalism in Queer Times* (Durham, NC: Duke University Press, 2007).

77. David Eng, *The Feeling of Kinship: Queer Liberalism and the Racialization of Intimacy* (Durham, NC: Duke University Press, 2010), xi.

78. Ann Cvetkovich, *An Archive of Feelings* (Durham, NC: Duke University Press, 2003), 11. Also see: Heather Love, *Feeling Backward: Loss and the Politics of Queer History* (Cambridge, MA: Harvard University Press, 2007), 21; Jack Halberstam, *The Queer Art of Failure* (Durham, NC: Duke University Press, 2011), for example 94–96.

79. Sara Ahmed, *The Promise of Happiness* (Durham, NC: Duke University Press, 2010); Halberstam, *The Queer Art of Failure*.

80. Halberstam, *The Queer Art of Failure*, 3.

81. Halberstam, *The Queer Art of Failure*; Ahmed, *The Promise of Happiness*; Eng, *The Feeling of Kinship*; Love, *Feeling Backward*.

## NOTES TO CHAPTER 3

1. Jessica Fields, "'Children Having Children': Race, Innocence, and Sexuality Education," *Social Problems* 52, no. 4 (2005): 550.

2. Rubin, "Thinking Sex," 282.

3. Nelson, *The Argonauts*.

4. Solanas, "SCUM Manifesto."

5. Opie, *Self-Portrait/Nursing* and *Self-Portrait/Cutting*; Shraya, *Trisha*.

6. José Esteban Muñoz, "Feeling Brown: Ethnicity and Affect in Ricardo Bracho's *The Sweetest Hangover (and Other STDs)*," *Theatre Journal* 52, no. 1 (2000): 67–79.

7. Warner, *The Trouble with Normal*, 217. Warner makes this statement in his discussion of the politics of shame in regard to HIV/AIDS, arguing against the politics of sexual aversion used to curb the spread of the virus. He goes on to say, "Gay men cannot be expected to eliminate their unconscious. They cannot be expected to live asexual lives." *The Trouble with Normal*, 218.

8. Barounis, "Compulsory Sexuality and Asexual/Crip Resistance," 175, 184.

9. M. Milks, "Stunted Growth: Asexual Politics and the Rhetoric of Sexual Liberation," in *Asexualities: Feminist and Queer Perspectives*, ed. KJ Cerankowski and M. Milks (New York: Routledge, 2014), 101.

10. Jake Pyne, "Arresting Ashley X: Trans Youth, Puberty Blockers and the Question of Whether Time Is on Your Side," *Somatechnics* 7, no. 1 (2017): 96–97.

11. Valerie Rohy, *Anachronism and Its Others: Sexuality, Race, Temporality* (New York: SUNY Press, 2009).

12. Ela Przybylo and Polina Ivleva, "Teaching It Straight: Sexuality Education across Post-State-Socialist Contexts," in *Childhood and Schooling in (Post)Socialist Societies: Memories of Everyday Life,* ed. Iveta Silova, Nelli Piattoeva, and Zsuzsa Millei (London: Palgrave Macmillan, 2018), 183–203.

13. Fields, "Children Having Children," 560.

14. Roberts, *Killing the Black Body,* 21. Also see Henry Giroux, *Stealing Innocence: Youth, Corporate Power, and the Politics of Culture* (New York: St. Martin's Press, 2000).

15. Robyn Maynard, *Policing Black Lives: State Violence in Canada from Slavery to the Present* (Black Point: Fernwood Publishing, 2017).

16. Robin Bernstein, *Racial Innocence: Performing American Childhood from Slavery to Civil Rights* (New York: New York University Press, 2011), 41.

17. Ta-Nehisi Coates, *Between the World and Me* (New York City: Spiegel and Grau, 2015).

18. Eve Tuck and K. Wayne Yang, "Decolonization Is Not a Metaphor," *Decolonization: Indigeneity, Education & Society* 1, no. 1 (2012): 3. They draw on a thesis by Janet Lee Mawhinney, "'Giving up the Ghost': Disrupting the (Re)production of White Privilege in Anti-racist Pedagogy and Organizational Change" (Master's Thesis, Ontario Institute for Studies in Education of the University of Toronto, 1998).

19. Hawkins Owen, "On the Racialization of Asexuality."

20. Barrie Thorne, "Re-Visioning Women and Social Change: Where Are the Children?" *Gender and Society* 1, no. 1 (1987): 85–109.

21. Pyne, "Arresting Ashley X"; Alison Kafer, *Feminist, Queer, Crip* (Bloomington: Indiana University Press, 2013).

22. Jacob Breslow, "*The Theory and Practice of Childhood: Interrogating Childhood as a Technology of Power*" (PhD thesis, London School of Economics and Political Science, 2016), 12.

23. Bracha Ettinger, *The Matrixial Borderspace* (Minneapolis: University of Minnesota Press, 2005). See also Susan (Contratto) Weisskopf, "Maternal Sexuality and Asexual Motherhood," *Signs: Journal of Women in Culture and Society* 5, no. 4 (1980): 766–82.

24. Freud, *Three Essays on the Theory of Sexuality.*

25. Freud, *Three Essays on the Theory of Sexuality,* 57.

26. Freud, *Three Essays on the Theory of Sexuality,* 57.

27. Freud, "Female Sexuality."

28. Nettie Pollard, "The Small Matter of Children," in *Bad Girls and Dirty Pictures: The Challenge to Reclaim Feminism,* ed. Alison Assiter and Avedon Carol (London: Pluto, 1993); Cristina L. H. Traina, *Erotic Attunement: Parenthood and the Ethics of Sensuality between Unequals* (Chicago: University of Chicago Press, 2011); Weisskopf, "Maternal Sexuality and Asexual Motherhood."

29. Sedgwick, *Tendencies,* 2, 3.

30. José Esteban Muñoz, *Cruising Utopia: The Then and There of Queer Futurity* (New York: New York University Press, 2009), 94; Kafer, *Feminist, Queer, Crip,* 31–33; Simon D. Elin Fisher, Rasheedah Phillips, and Ido H. Katri, "Trans Temporalities (Introduction to Special Issue)," *Somatechnics* 7, no. 1 (2017): 1–15.

31. Ellen Samuels, "Cripping Anti-Futurity, or, If You Love Queer Theory So Much, Why Don't You Marry It?'" in *Annual Meeting of Society for Disability Studies* (San Jose, California, June 15–18, 2011).

32. Steven Angelides, "Feminism, Child Sexual Abuse, and the Erasure of Child Sexuality," *GLQ: A Journal of Lesbian and Gay Studies* 10, no. 2 (2004): 141–77.

33. Angelides, "Feminism, Child Sexual Abuse, and the Erasure of Child Sexuality," 142.

34. Angelides, "Feminism, Child Sexual Abuse, and the Erasure of Child Sexuality," 146, 155, 166, 162.

35. Rubin, "Thinking Sex," 278.

36. Annamarie Jagose, "Counterfeit Pleasures: Fake Orgasm and Queer Agency," *Textual Practice* 24, no. 3 (2010): 517. Also see Leo Bersani, "Is the Rectum a Grave?" *October* 43 (1987): 197–222; Yasmin Nair, "Your Sex Is Not Radical," June 7, 2015, http://yasminnair.net/content/your-sex-not-radical.

37. Bersani, "Is the Rectum a Grave?," 205.

38. Nair, "Your Sex Is Not Radical."

39. Bersani, "Is the Rectum a Grave?," 206.

40. Jagose, "Counterfeit Pleasures."

41. Jagose, "Counterfeit Pleasures," 518.

42. Karín Lesnik-Oberstein, "Childhood, Queer Theory, and Feminism," *Feminist Theory* 11, no. 3 (2010): 315.

43. Nelson, *The Argonauts*.

44. Nelson, *The Argonauts*.

45. Nelson, *The Argonauts*, 5, 28.

46. Przybylo and Cooper, "Asexual Resonances"; Opie, *Self-Portrait/Nursing* and *Self-Portrait/Cutting*.

47. Nelson, *The Argonauts*. Dick Blau, *Observations of a Mother*, 1986–1997. See Jane Gallop, "Observations of a Mother," in *The Familial Gaze*, ed. Marianne Hirsch (Hanover, NH: Dartmouth College, 1999); Susan Fraiman, *Cool Men and the Second Sex* (New York: Columbia University Press, 2003), 134; Sigmund Freud, *The "Wolf" Man* (1918), trans. Louise Adey Huish (London, Penguin Books, 1918/2002); A. L. Steiner, *Puppies and Babies*, University of Southern California, 3001 Gallery, 2012.

48. Nelson, *The Argonauts*, 72.

49. Fraiman, *Cool Men and the Second Sex*.

50. Donald Winnicott, *The Family and Individual Development* (London: Tavistock Publications, 1965).

51. Nelson, *The Argonauts*, 20.

52. Nelson, *The Argonauts*, 44.

53. Nelson, *The Argonauts*, 42.

54. Donald Winnicott quoted in Nelson, *The Argonauts*, 142.

55. Nelson, *The Argonauts*, 98.

56. Nelson, *The Argonauts*, 73.

57. Nelson, *The Argonauts*, 110.

58. Solanas, "SCUM," 213.

59. Breanne Fahs, "The Radical Possibilities of Valerie Solanas," *Feminist Studies* 34, no. 3 (2008): 598.

60. Kim, "Asexualities and Disabilities in Constructing Sexual Normalcy"; Gupta, "Compulsory Sexuality."

61. Milks, "Stunted Growth," 101.

62. Nelson, *The Argonauts*, 111.

63. Nelson, *The Argonauts*, 110. Solanas, "SCUM," 213. See Barounis, "Compulsory Sexuality and Asexual/Crip Resistance."

64. Nelson, *The Argonauts*, 110–111.

65. For Opie's artwork, visit https://artsandculture.google.com/asset/self-portrait-nursing/SgHoN6WNo_B8gw and https://artsandculture.google.com/asset/self-portrait-cutting/yQG2x2FpePzJXw.

66. Bernstein, *Racial Innocence*, 39; Ettinger, *The Matrixial Borderspace*; Barbara Sichtermann, "The Lost Eroticism of the Breasts," in *Femininity: The Politics of the Personal* (Minneapolis: University of Minnesota Press, 1986), 57; Traina, *Erotic Attunement*; Weisskopf, "Maternal Sexuality and Asexual Motherhood."

67. Roberts, *Killing the Black Body*, 179.

68. Roberts, *Killing the Black Body*, 208.

69. James Kincaid, *Erotic Innocence* (Durham, NC: Duke University Press, 1998); Roberts, Killing the Black Body; Ann Laura Stoler, *Race and the Education of Desire* (Durham, NC: Duke University Press, 1995).
70. Hawkins Owen, "On the Racialization of Asexuality," 122.
71. Hawkins Owen, "On the Racialization of Asexuality," 127. Charles W. Mills, *The Racial Contract* (Ithaca, NY: Cornell University Press, 1997).
72. Hawkins Owen, "On the Racialization of Asexuality," 121. See also Carter, *The Heart of Whiteness.*
73. Opie, *Self-Portrait/Nursing* and *Self-Portrait/Cutting.*
74. Opie, *Self-Portrait/Cutting.*
75. Opie, *Self-Portrait/Nursing.*
76. Amy Adler, "The Perverse Law of Child Pornography," *Columbia Law Review* 101, no. 2 (2001): 256.
77. Nelson, *The Argonauts,* 64.
78. Shraya, *Trisha.*
79. Kathryn Bond Stockton, *The Queer Child, or, Growing Sideways in the Twentieth Century* (Durham, NC: Duke University Press, 2009), 4.
80. Clementine Morrigan, "Trauma Time: The Queer Temporalities of the Traumatized Mind," *Somatechnics* 7, no. 1 (2017): 50–58.
81. Muñoz, "Feeling Brown."
82. Sheila L. Cavanagh, "Trans* Photography, Sexual Difference and the m/Other in Vivek Shraya's *Trisha,*" Sexuality Studies Association (Toronto: Ryerson University, May 28, 2017), 3. Available online at http://sheila.info.yorku.ca/keynotes-and-public-presentations/. See also Ettinger, *The Matrixial Borderspace.*
83. Elizabeth Freeman, *Time Binds: Queer Temporalities, Queer Histories* (Durham, NC: Duke University Press, 2010) 59.
84. Weisskopf, "Maternal Sexuality and Asexual Motherhood," 773.
85. Huffer, *Are the Lips a Grave?*; Lorde, "The Uses of the Erotic."
86. Kincaid, *Erotic Innocence,* 14.
87. Steven Bruhm and Natasha Hurley, *Curiouser: On the Queerness of Children* (Minneapolis: University of Minnesota Press, 2004), xxx; Sara Ahmed, *Queer Phenomenology: Orientations, Objects, Others* (Durham, NC: Duke University Press, 2006).
88. Kincaid, *Erotic Innocence,* 14.
89. Kincaid, *Erotic Innocence,* 14.
90. Kincaid, *Erotic Innocence,* 24.
91. Kincaid, *Erotic Innocence,* 24.

## NOTES TO CHAPTER 4

1. Monica J. Casper and Lisa Jean Moore, *Missing Bodies: The Politics of Visibility* (New York: New York University Press, 2009).
2. Stephen Katz, "Hold On! Falling, Embodiment, and the Materiality of Old Age," in *Corpus,* ed. Monica J. Casper and Paisley Currah (New York: Palgrave Macmillan, 2011), 187.
3. Susan Wendell has talked about aging in relation to disability in *The Rejected Body: Feminist Philosophical Reflections on Disability* (New York: Routledge, 1996). Also see Elizabeth Lightfoot, "Disability," *Handbook of Gerontology: Evidence-Based Approaches to Theory, Practice, and Policy,* ed. James A. Blackburn and Catherine N. Dulmus (Hoboken, NJ: John Wiley and Sons, 2007); Meredith Minkler and Pamela Fadem, "'Successful Aging': A Disability Perspective," *Journal of Disability Policy Studies* 12, no. 4 (2002): 229–35.

4. Kafer, *Feminist, Queer, Crip,* 23.

5. Coviello, *Tomorrow's Parties*; Trisha Franzen, *Spinsters and Lesbians: Independent Womanhood in the United States* (New York: New York University Press, 1996); Amy Froide, *Never Married: Singlewomen in Early Modern England* (Oxford: Oxford University Press, 2005); Bridget Hill, *Women Alone: Spinsters in England 1660–1850* (New Haven, CT: Yale University Press, 2001); Kahan, *Celibacies*; Kent, *Making Girls into Women*; Heather Love, "Gyn/Apology: Sarah Orne Jewett's Spinster Aesthetics," *ESQ: A Journal of American Renaissance* 55, no. 3–4 (2009): 305–34; Davida Pines, *The Marriage Paradox: Modernist Novels and the Cultural Imperative to Marry* (Gainesville: University of Florida Press, 2006).

6. Love, "Gyn/Apology," 329; Hannah McGregor, "The Loneliness of the Spinster," *Chronicle Vitae,* 2016, https://chroniclevitae.com/news/1609-the-loneliness-of-the-spinster.

7. Froide, *Never Married*.

8. Dana Luciano, *Arranging Grief: Sacred Time and the Body in Nineteenth-Century* (New York: New York University Press, 2007), 9.

9. Giorgio Agamben, *Homo Sacer: Sovereign Power and Bare Life,* trans. Daniel Heller-Roazen (Stanford, CA: Stanford University Press, 1998); Foucault, *The History of Sexuality*; Ranjana Khanna, "Disposability," *differences: A Journal of Feminist Cultural Studies* 20, no. 1 (2009): 181–98.

10. Baumbach, *Frances Ha*.

11. Foucault, *The History of Sexuality,* 139.

12. Michel Foucault, "Lecture Eleven: 17 March 1976," in *Society Must Be Defended: Lectures at the College de France, 1975–1976* (New York: Picador, 2003), 251. See also Achille Mbembe, "Necropolitics," *Public Culture* 15, no. 1 (2003): 11–40.

13. Angela Davis, "Racism, Birth Control, and Reproductive Rights," in *Women, Race, and Class* (New York: Vintage Books, 1983), 221.

14. Agamben, *Homo Sacer,* 28.

15. Khanna, "Disposability," 182, 184, 186.

16. Khanna, "Disposability," 186, 190.

17. Foucault, *The History of Sexuality*.

18. Paul Simpson, Maria Horne, Laura J. E. Brown, Christine Brown Wilson, Tommy Dickinson, and Kate Torkington, "Old(er) Care Home Residents and Sexual/Intimate Citizenship," *Ageing and Society* 37, no. 2 (2016): 10.

19. Simpson et al., "Old(er) Care Home Residents and Sexual/Intimate Citizenship," 1.

20. Evelyn Reynolds, "In America, Aging while Black Takes Solidarity, Activism and Magic," *Huffpost,* 2017, https://www.huffingtonpost.com/entry/aging-while-black-activism_us_58a477efe4b094a129f106eb.

21. Geniece Crawford Mondé, "#BlackDontCrack: A Content Analysis of the Aging Black Woman in Social Media," *Feminist Media Studies* 18, no. 1 (2018): 47–60.

22. Ruth Wilson Gilmore, *Golden Gulag: Prisons, Surplus, Crisis, and Opposition in Globalizing California* (Berkeley: University of California Press, 2007), 28.

23. Hawkins Owen, "On the Racialization of Asexuality," 125.

24. Linda J. Brock and Glen Jennings, "Sexuality and Intimacy," in *Handbook of Gerontology: Evidence-Based Approaches to Theory, Practice, and Policy,* ed. James A. Blackburn and Catherine N. Dulmus (Hoboken, NJ: John Wiley and Sons, 2007), 244.

25. Lynne Segal, *Out of Time: The Pleasures and Perils of Aging* (London: Verso, 2014), 2.

26. Melissa Muehlbauer and Patricia Crane, "Elder Abuse and Neglect," *Journal of Psychosocial Nursing and Mental Health Services* 44, no. 11 (2006): 43–48; Linda R. Phillips, Guifang Guo, and Haesook Kim, "Elder Mistreatment in U. S. Residential Care Facilities: The Scope of the Problem," *Journal of Elder Abuse & Neglect* 25, no. 1 (2013): 19–39.

27. Katherine E. Bradway and Renée L. Beard, "'Don't Be Trying to Box Folks In': Older Women's Sexuality," *Affilia: Journal of Women and Social Work* 20, no. 4 (2015): 512.

28. Emily Waterman, "Reactions of College Students to the Sexuality of Older People," *Journal of Student Research* 1, no. 2 (2012): 46–50.

29. Mally Ehrenfeld, Nili Tabak, Gila Bronner, and Rebecca Bergman, "Ethical Dilemmas Concerning the Sexuality of Elderly Patients Suffering from Dementia," *International Journal of Nursing Practice* 3, no. 4 (1997): 255–59.

30. Michelle Meagher, "Jenny Saville and a Feminist Aesthetics of Disgust," *Hypatia* 18, no. 4 (2003): 24.

31. Hilde Lindemann Nelson, "Stories of My Old Age," in *Mother Time: Women, Aging, Ethics*, ed. Margaret Urban Walker (New York: Rowman and Littlefield, 2000), 89.

32. Jane M. Ussher, *Managing the Monstrous Feminine: Regulating the Reproductive Body* (London: Routledge, 2006).

33. Susan Wendell, "Old Women Out of Control: Some Thoughts on Aging, Ethics, and Psychosomatic Medicine," in *Mother Time: Women, Aging, Ethics*, ed. Margaret Urban Walker, (New York: Rowman and Littlefield, 2000), 135.

34. Mary Douglas, *Purity and Danger: An Analysis of the Concepts of Pollution and Taboo* (London: Routledge and Kegan Paul, 1966); Julia Kristeva, *The Powers of Horror: An Essay on Abjection*, trans. Leon S. Roudiez (New York: Columbia University Press, 1982); Meagher, "Jenny Saville and a Feminist Aesthetics of Disgust."

35. Erving Goffman, *Asylums: Essays on the Social Situation of Mental Patients and Other Inmates* (Garden City, NY: Anchor Books, 1961), xiii.

36. Goffman, *Asylums*, 6, 7.

37. Tove Persson and David Wästerfors, "'Such Trivial Matters': How Staff Account for Restrictions of Residents' Influence in Nursing Homes," *Journal of Aging Studies* 23, no. 1 (2009): 8.

38. Goffman, *Asylums*, 11.

39. Goffman, *Asylums*, 11.

40. Simpson et al., "Old(er) Care Home Residents and Sexual/Intimate Citizenship," 9.

41. Persson and Wästerfors, "Such Trivial Matters," 6.

42. Ann-Mari Sellerberg, "Expressivity within a Time Schedule: Subordinated Interaction on Geriatric Wards," *Sociology of Health and Illness* 13, no. 1 (1991): 69.

43. Sabine Pleschberger, "Dignity and the Challenge of Dying in Nursing Homes: The Residents' View," *Age and Ageing* 36, no. 2 (2007): 199; Bradway and Beard, "Don't Be Trying to Box Folks In," 511.

44. Joan C. Tronto, "Age-Segregated Housing As a Moral Problem: An Exercise in Rethinking Ethics," in *Mother Time: Women, Aging, Ethics*, ed. Margaret Urban Walker (New York: Rowman and Littlefield, 2000), 262.

45. Goffman, *Asylums*, 6.

46. Sharon Hinchliff and Marryn Gott, "Challenging Social Myths and Stereotypes of Women and Aging: Heterosexual Women Talk about Sex," *Journal of Women and Aging* 20, no. 1/2 (2008): 65–81.

47. Yulia Watters and Tommie V. Boyd, "Sexuality in Later Life: Opportunity for Reflections for Healthcare Providers," *Sexual and Relationship Therapy* 24, no. 3–4 (2009): 307.

48. Laci J. Cornelison and Gayle M. Doll, "Management of Sexual Expression in Long-Term Care: Ombudsmen's Perspectives," *The Gerontologist* 53, no. 5 (2012): 780–89; Susan Deacon, Victor Minichiello, and David Plummer, "Sexuality and Older People: Revisiting the Assumptions," *Educational Gerontology* 21, no. 5 (1995): 497; Simpson et al., "Old(er) Care Home Residents and Sexual/Intimate Citizenship," 16.

49. Rebec et al., "Breaking Down Taboos Concerning Sexuality among the Elderly."

50. Cornelison and Doll, "Management of Sexual Expression in Long-Term Care."

51. David Holmes, Jacob Reingold, and Jeanne Teresi, "Sexual Expression and Dementia. Views of Caregivers: A Pilot Study," *International Journal of Geriatric Psychiatry* 12, no. 7 (1997): 696–701.

52. Cornelison and Doll, "Management of Sexual Expression in Long-Term Care."

53. Lauren Breland, "Lost Libido, or Just Forgotten? The Legal and Social Influences on Sexual Activity in Long-Term Care," *Law and Psychology Review* 38 (2014): 177–92; Kristin Scherrer, "Images of Sexuality and Aging in Gerontological Literature," *Sexuality Research and Social Policy* 6, no. 4 (2009): 5–12.

54. Anna Siverskog, "Ageing Bodies That Matter: Age, Gender and Embodiment in Older Transgender People's Life Stories," *NORA: Nordic Journal of Feminist and Gender Research* 23, no. 1 (2015): 4–19.

55. Mary Beth Foglia and Karen I. Fredriksen-Goldsen, "Health Disparities among LGBT Older Adults and the Role of Nonconscious Bias," *LGBT Bioethics: Visibility, Disparities, and Dialogue,* special report, *Hastings Center Report* 44, no. 5 (2014): S40–S44; Joy Phillips and Genée Marks, "Ageing Lesbians: Marginalizing Discourses and Social Exclusion in the Aged Care Industry," *Journal of Lesbian and Gay Social Services* 20, no. 1/2 (2008): 187–202.

56. Segal, *Out of Time,* 227.

57. Watters and Boyd, "Sexuality in Later Life," 310.

58. Margaret Hellie Huyck, "Romantic Relationship in Later Life," *Generations* 25, no. 2 (2001): 9–17.

59. Sheyna Sears-Roberts Alterovits and Gerald A. Mendelsohn, "Partner Preferences across the Life Span: Online Dating by Older Adults," *Psychology and Aging* 24, no. 2 (2009): 513–17. See also Deacon, Minichiello, and Plummer, "Sexuality and Older People," 499.

60. Vanessa Denardi Antoniassi Baldissera, Sonia Maria Villela Bueno, and Luiza Akiko Komura Hoga, "Improvement of Older Women's Sexuality through Emancipatory Education," *Health Care for Women International* 33, no. 10 (2012): 956–72; Deacon, Minichiello, and Plummer, "Sexuality and Older People," 499; John DeLamater and Morgan Sill, "Sexual Desire in Later Life," *The Journal of Sex Research* 42, no. 2 (2005): 138–49; Victor Minichiello, David Plummer, and Anne Seal, "The 'Asexual' Older Person? Australian Evidence," *Venereology* 9, no. 3 (1996): 180–88.

61. James Wilkins, "More Than Capacity: Alternatives for Sexual Decision Making for Individuals with Dementia," *The Gerontologist* 55, no. 5 (2015): 716–73.

62. Breland in "Lost Libido, or Just Forgotten?" looks at Alabama.

63. Wilkins, "More Than Capacity," 719.

64. Such as in Wisconsin; see Breland, "Lost Libido, or Just Forgotten?," 184.

65. Lightfoot, "Disability," 202.

66. Shaka McGlotten and Lisa Jean Moore, "The Geriatric Clinic: Dry and Limp: Aging Queers, Zombies, and Sexual Reanimation," *Journal of Medical Humanities* 34, no. 2 (2013): 261–68.

67. Simpson et al., "Old(er) Care Home Residents and Sexual/Intimate Citizenship," 4, 9.

68. Kim, "Asexualities and Disabilities in Constructing Sexual Normalcy"; Kim, "How Much Sex Is Healthy?"; Lund and Johnson, "Asexuality and Disability."

69. Bradway and Beard, "Don't Be Trying to Box Folks In," 504–5.

70. Bradway and Beard, "Don't Be Trying to Box Folks In," 504.

71. Waterman, "Reactions of College Students to the Sexuality of Older People," 46.

72. Simpson et al., "Old(er) Care Home Residents and Sexual/Intimate Citizenship," 4.

73. Stephen Katz and Barbara Marshall, "New Sex for Old: Lifestyle, Consumerism, and the Ethics of Aging Well," *Journal of Aging Studies* 17, no. 1 (2003): 13, 4.

74. Stephen Katz and Barbara Marshall, "Forever Functional: Sexual Fitness and the Ageing Male Body," *Body & Society* 8, no. 4 (2002): 43–70; Meika Loe, "Sex and the Senior Woman: Pleasure and Danger in the Viagra Era," *Sexualities* 7, no. 3 (2004): 303–36; Annie Potts, Nicola Gavey, Victoria M. Grace, and Tiina Vares, "The Downside of Viagra: Women's Experiences and Concerns," *Sociology of Health & Illness* 25, no. 1 (2003): 697–719.

75. McGlotten and Moore, "The Geriatric Clinic," 261.

76. Katz and Marshall, "New Sex for Old." See also Jonathan M. Metzl and Anna Kirkland, eds., *Against Health: How Health Became the New Morality* (New York: New York University Press, 2010).

77. Edmonds, "Surgery-for-Life," 249.

78. John Rowe and Robert Kahn, "Successful Aging," *The Gerontologist* 37, no. 4 (1997): 433–40; Thomas Cole, *The Journey of Life: A Cultural History of Aging in America* (Cambridge: Cambridge University Press, 1992), 239.

79. Edmonds, "Surgery-for-Life," 254.

80. Katz and Marshall, "Forever Functional," 55.

81. Hinchliff and Gott, "Challenging Social Myths and Stereotypes of Women and Aging," 67; Merryn Gott and Sharron Hinchliff, "How Important Is Sex in Later Life? The Views of Older People," *Social Science and Medicine* 56 (2003): 1618.

82. Marryn Gott, *Sexuality, Sexual Health and Ageing* (Berkshire: Open University Press, 2005). Also see Gupta, "Screw Health."

83. Brock and Jennings, "Sexuality and Intimacy," 251; Deacon, Minichiello, and Plummer, "Sexuality and Older People," 498.

84. Watters and Boyd, "Sexuality in Later Life," 312; Deacon, Minichiello, and Plummer, "Sexuality and Older People," 498.

85. Brock and Jennings, "Sexuality and Intimacy," 244, 251; Deacon, Minichiello, and Plummer, "Sexuality and Older People"; Watters and Boyd, "Sexuality in Later Life," 312; Wilkins, "More Than Capacity," 716.

86. Sandra Lee Bartky, "Unplanned Obsolescence: Some Reflections on Aging," in *Mother Time: Women, Aging, Ethics*, ed. Margaret Urban Walker (New York: Rowman and Littlefield, 2000), 72–73.

87. Warner, *The Trouble with Normal*, 139, 115–116.

88. Bartky, "Unplanned Obsolescence."

89. Bartky, "Unplanned Obsolescence," 72.

90. Bartky, "Unplanned Obsolescence," 73.

91. Bartky, "Unplanned Obsolescence," 73.

92. Bolick, *Spinster*; McGregor, "The Loneliness of the Spinster."

93. Mary Daly, *Gyn/Ecology: The Metaethics of Radical Feminism* (Boston: Beacon Press, 1978/1990); Rich, "Compulsory Heterosexuality."

94. Quoted in Love, "Gyn/Apology." Daly, *Gyn/Ecology*, 1. For a list of feminists who draw on the spinster figure for inspiration, see Love, "Gyn/Apology," 330fn3.

95. Coviello, *Tomorrow's Parties*; Franzen, *Spinsters and Lesbians*; Froide, *Never Married*; Hill, *Women Alone*; Kahan, *Celibacies*; Kent, *Making Girls into Women*; Love, "Gyn/Apology"; Pines, *The Marriage Paradox*.

96. Froide, *Never Married*, 1.

97. Froide, *Never Married*, 1–14, 155; Hill, *Women Alone*, 4.

98. Kent, *Making Girls into Women*, 24.

99. Kent, *Making Girls into Women*, 21. Hortense Spillers, "Interstices: A Small Drama of Words," in *Pleasure and Danger: Exploring Female Sexuality*, ed. Carole S. Vance (London: Routledge and Kegan Paul, 1984), 73–100. Also see Kahan, *Celibacies*, 94.

100. Sheila L. Cavanagh, *Sexing the Teacher: School Sex Scandals and Queer Pedagogies* (Vancouver: University of British Columbia Press, 2007); Kent, *Making Girls into Women*.

101. Kent, *Making Girls into Women*, 34–35.

102. Rita Kranidis, *The Victorian Spinster and Colonial Emigration: Contested Subjects* (New York: St. Martin's Press, 1999), 4–5, 173–180.

103. Cavanagh, *Sexing the Teacher*, 7.

104. Cobb, *Single*, 8, 31.

105. Luna, "Romantic Love Is Killing Us."

106. Eleanor Wilkinson, "The Romantic Imaginary: Compulsory Coupledom and Single Existence," in *Sexualities: Past Reflections, Future Directions*, ed. Sally Hines and Yvette Taylor (London: Palgrave Macmillan, 2012), 130–45.

107. Berlant, *Cruel Optimism*; Sarah Carter, *The Importance of Being Monogamous: Marriage and Nation Building in Western Canada to 1915* (Edmonton: University of Alberta Press, 2008).

108. Mark Rifkin, *When Did Indians Become Straight? Kinship, the History of Sexuality, and Native Sovereignty* (New York: Oxford University Press, 2011).

109. Love, "Gyn/Apology"; Warner, *The Trouble with Normal*.

110. Kahan, *Celibacies*, 74.

111. Coviello, *Tomorrow's Parties*, 4.

112. Doan, introduction to *Old Maids to Radical Spinsters: Unmarried Women in the Twentieth Century Novel*, ed. Laura Doan (Urbana: University of Illinois Press, 1991), 4.

113. Nina Auerbach, foreword in *Old Maids to Radical Spinsters: Unmarried Women in the Twentieth-Century Novel*, ed. Laura Doan (Urbana: University of Illinois Press, 1991), xiv.

114. Stockton, *The Queer Child*. Jack Halberstam, *In a Queer Time and Place* (New York: New York University Press, 2005).

115. Simon Dickel, "Between Mumblecore and Post-Black Aesthetics: Barry Jenkins's *Medicine for Melancholy*," in *Understanding Blackness through Performance: Contemporary Arts and the Representation of Identity*, ed. Anne Crémieux, Xavier Lemoine, and Jean-Paul Rocchi (Basingstoke: Palgrave Macmillan, 2013), 109–23.

116. Coviello, *Tomorrow's Parties*, 11.

117. Coviello, *Tomorrow's Parties*, 11.

118. Muñoz, *Cruising Utopia*.

119. Baumbach, *Frances Ha*.

120. Baumbach, *Frances Ha*.

121. Baumbach, *Frances Ha*.

122. Baumbach, *Frances Ha*.

123. Baumbach, *Frances Ha*.

124. Annamarie Jagose, *Orgasmology* (Durham, NC: Duke University Press, 2013).

125. Coviello, *Tomorrow's Parties*, 4.

126. Frantz Fanon, *Black Skin, White Masks*, trans. Richard Philcox (New York: Grove Press, 1952/2008); Jacques Lacan, "The Split between the Eye and the Gaze," in *The Four Fundamental Concepts of Psychoanalysis. The Seminar of Jacques Lacan*, Book 11, trans. Alan Sheridan (London: W. W. Norton, 1981), 72.

127. bell hooks, "The Oppositional Gaze: Black Female Spectators," in *Black Looks: Race and Representation* (Boston: South End Press, 1992), 115–31.

128. Berlant, *Cruel Optimism*.

129. Baumbach, *Frances Ha*. Freeman, *Time Binds*; Muñoz, *Cruising Utopia*.

130. Ahmed, *Queer Phenomenology*, 65–107.

131. Ahmed, *Queer Phenomenology*, 65–107.

132. Esther D. Rothblum, "Early Memories, Current Realities," in *Boston Marriages: Romantic but Asexual Relationships among Contemporary Lesbians*, ed. Esther D. Rothblum and Kathleen A. Brehony (Amherst: University of Massachusetts Press, 1993), 14.

133. Shannon Bell, *Fast Feminism* (New York: Automedia, 2010), 21.

## NOTES TO EPILOGUE

1. Minassian posted on his Facebook page: "We will overthrow all the Chads and Stacys! All hail the Supreme Gentleman Elliot Rodger!" Elliot Rodger killed six people and injured fourteen in 2014 at the University of California, Santa Barbara and wrote a mani-

festo titled "My Twisted World: The Story of Elliot Rodger" in which he discussed how he was denied sex by women. The manifesto is available online: https://www.document-cloud.org/documents/1173808-elliot-rodger-manifesto.html.

2. Note that the site itself does not condone violence against women or murderous rampages.

3. Casey Ryan Kelly, "Elliot Rodger's Retribution: The Thanatopolitics of Involuntary Celibacy," forthcoming. Elliot Rodger, "My Twisted World: The Story of Elliot Rodger," 2014, https://www.documentcloud.org/documents/1173808-elliot-rodger-manifesto.html.

4. Rodger, "My Twisted World," 84.

5. Rodger, "My Twisted World," 136.

6. Erin Spampinato, "The Literary Roots of the Incel Movement," *Electric Lit,* May 24, 2018, https://electricliterature.com/the-literary-roots-of-the-incel-movement-4ba183b9c9c5.

7. Lorde, "Uses of the Erotic," 55.

8. Peter Baker, "The Woman Who Accidentally Started the Incel Movement," *Elle,* March 2016, https://www.elle.com/culture/news/amp34512/woman-who-started-incel-movement/.

9. Rodger, "My Twisted World," 136.

# BIBLIOGRAPHY

Agamben, Giorgio. *Homo Sacer: Sovereign Power and Bare Life.* Translated by Daniel Heller-Roazen. Stanford, CA: Stanford University Press, 1998.

Ahmed, Sara. "Killing Joy: Feminism and the History of Happiness." *Signs: Journal of Women in Culture and Society* 35, no. 3 (2010): 571–94.

———. *The Promise of Happiness.* Durham, NC: Duke University Press, 2010.

———. *Queer Phenomenology: Orientations, Objects, Others.* Durham, NC: Duke University Press, 2006.

Aicken, Catherine, Catherine Mercer, and Jackie Cassell. "Who Reports Absence of Sexual Attraction in Britain? Evidence from National Probability Surveys." *Psychology & Sexuality* 4, no. 2 (2013): 121–35.

Allen, Indra. "Why I Am Celibate (Interview with Indra Allen by Dana Densmore)." *No More Fun and Games* 6 (1972/1973): 39–46.

American Psychiatric Association. *Diagnostic and Statistical Manual of Mental Disorders.* 3rd ed., rev. Washington, DC: APA, 1980.

———. *Diagnostic and Statistical Manual of Mental Disorders.* 4th ed. Washington, DC: American Psychiatric Press, 1994.

———. *Diagnostic and Statistical Manual of Mental Disorders.* 5th ed. Arlington, VA: American Psychiatric Publishing, 2013.

Angelides, Steven. "Feminism, Child Sexual Abuse, and the Erasure of Child Sexuality." *GLQ: A Journal of Lesbian and Gay Studies* 10, no. 2 (2004): 141–77.

Antoniassi Baldissera, Vanessa Denardi, Sonia Maria Villela Bueno, and Luiza Akiko Komura Hoga. "Improvement of Older Women's Sexuality through Emancipatory Education." *Health Care for Women International* 33, no. 10 (2012): 956–72.

"A Record of 'Lesbian Bedrooms': An Interview with Photographer Kyle Lasky–NMP." *No More Potlucks* 22 (2012). http://nomorepotlucks.org/site/record-lesbian-bedrooms/.

Asexual Awareness Week Team and Tristan Miller (aka Siggy). "Asexual Community Census 2011" (2011). http:/ fasexualawarenessweek.comfdocsfSiggyAnalysis-AAWCensus.pdf.

Atkinson, Ti-Grace. "The Institution of Sexual Intercourse." In *Notes from the Second Year: Women's Liberation,* 42–47. New York: New York Radical Feminists, 1970.

———. "Lesbianism and Feminism: Justice for Women as 'Unnatural.'" In *Amazon Odyssey: The First Collection of Writings by the Political Pioneer of the Women's Movement*, 131–34. New York: Link Books, 1970/1974.

———. "Radical Feminism and Love." In *Amazon Odyssey: The First Collection of Writings by the Political Pioneer of the Women's Movement*, 41–45. New York: Link Books, 1969/1974.

Auerbach, Nina. Foreword in *Old Maids to Radical Spinsters: Unmarried Women in the Twentieth-Century Novel*, edited by Laura Doan, ix–xv. Urbana: University of Illinois Press, 1991.

AVEN: Asexual Visibility and Education Network. 2001–2012. https://www.asexuality.org.

Avenwiki. "Lexicon." http://wiki.asexuality.org/Lexicon.

Awkward-Rich, Cameron. "A Prude's Manifesto." *Button Poetry*, 2015. https://www.facebook.com/ButtonPoetry/videos/1277265262331016/?hc_ref=PAGES_TIMELINE.

Baker, Peter. "The Woman Who Accidentally Started the Incel Movement." *Elle*, March 2016. https://www.elle.com/culture/news/amp34512/woman-who-started-incel-movement/.

Bambara, Toni Cade. "On the Issue of Roles." In *The Black Woman: An Anthology*, edited by Toni Cade Bambara, 101–10. New York: Washington Square Press, 1970.

———. "The Pill: Genocide or Liberation?" In *The Black Woman: An Anthology*, edited by Toni Cade Bambara, 162–69. New York: New American Library, 1970.

———. Preface to *The Black Woman: An Anthology*, edited by Toni Cade Bambara, 7–12. New York: New American Library, 1970.

Barker, Meg, and Darren Langdridge, eds. *Understanding Non-Monogamies*. London: Routledge, 2010.

Barounis, Cynthia. "Compulsory Sexuality and Asexual/Crip Resistance in John Cameron Mitchell's *Shortbus*." In *Asexualities: Feminist and Queer Perspectives*, edited by KJ Cerankowski and M. Milks, 174–96. New York: Routledge, 2014.

Bartky, Sandra Lee. "Unplanned Obsolescence: Some Reflections on Aging." In *Mother Time: Women, Aging, Ethics*, edited by Margaret Urban Walker, 61–74. New York: Rowman and Littlefield, 2000.

Batričević, Milica, and Andrej Cvetić. "Uncovering an A: Asexuality and Asexual Activism in Croatia and Serbia." In *Intersectionality and LGBT Activist Politics*, edited by Bojan Bilić and Sanja Kajinić, 77–103. London: Palgrave Macmillan, 2016.

Baumbach, Noah, dir. *Frances Ha*. New York: RT Features, 2012.

Beale, Frances. "Double Jeopardy: To Be Black and Female." In *The Black Woman: An Anthology*, edited by Toni Cade Bambara, 90–100. New York: New American Library, 1970.

Bear, Tracy. "Power in My Blood: Corporeal Sovereignty through the Praxis of an Indigenous Eroticanalysis." PhD diss., University of Alberta, 2016.

Beauvoir, Simone de. *The Second Sex*. New York: Vintage Books, 1949/2012.

Bechdel, Alison. *The Essential Dykes to Watch Out For*. Boston: Houghton Mifflin Harcourt, 2008.

Beirne, Rebecca. *Lesbians in Television and Text after the Millennium*. London: Palgrave Macmillan, 2008.

Bell, Shannon. *Fast Feminism*. New York: Automedia, 2010.

Bennett, Bob. "(Title)." In *Black Fire: An Anthology of Afro-American Writing*, edited by LeRoi Jones and Larry Neal, 423. New York: William Morrow, 1968.

Berlant, Lauren. *Cruel Optimism*. Durham, NC: Duke University Press, 2011.

Berlant, Lauren, and Lee Edelman. *Sex, or the Unbearable*. Durham, NC: Duke University Press, 2012.

Berlant, Lauren, and Michael Warner. "Sex in Public." *Critical Inquiry* 24, no. 2 (1998): 547–66.

Bernstein, Robin. *Racial Innocence: Performing American Childhood from Slavery to Civil Rights*. New York: New York University Press, 2011.

Bersani, Leo. "Is the Rectum a Grave?" *October* 43 (1987): 197–222.

Berson, Ginny. "The Furies." In *Lesbianism and the Women's Movement*, edited by The Furies, Nancy Myron, and Charlotte Bunch, 15–19. Baltimore: Diana Press, 1975.

———. "The Furies: Goddesses of Vengeance." *Serials Review* 16, no. 4 (1990): 79–87.

Blau, Dick. *Observations of a Mother*. 1986–1997.

Blumstein, Philip, and Pepper Schwartz. *American Couples: Money, Work, Sex*. New York: William Morrow, 1983.

Bogaert, Anthony. "Asexuality: Dysfunction or Variation?" In *Psychological Sexual Dysfunctions*, edited by Jayson M. Caroll and Marta K. Alena, 9–13. New York: Nova Science Publishers, 2008.

———. "Asexuality: Prevalence and Associated Factors in a National Probability Sample." *Journal of Sex Research* 41, no. 3 (2004): 279–87.

———. "Toward a Conceptual Understanding of Asexuality." *Review of General Psychology* 10, no. 3 (2006): 241–50.

———. *Understanding Asexuality*. Toronto: Rowman and Littlefield, 2012.

Bolick, Kate. *Spinster: Making a Life of One's Own*. New York: Pengiun, 2015.

Bond, Jean Carey, and Patricia Peery. "Is the Black Male Castrated?" In *The Black Woman: An Anthology*, edited by Toni Cade Bambara, 113–18. New York: New American Library, 1970.

Bradway, Katherine E., and Renée L. Beard. "'Don't Be Trying to Box Folks In': Older Women's Sexuality." *Affilia: Journal of Women and Social Work* 20, no. 4 (2015): 504–18.

Brake, Elizabeth. *Minimizing Marriage: Marriage, Morality, and the Law*. Oxford: Oxford University Press, 2012.

Breines, Winifred. *The Trouble between Us: An Uneasy History of White and Black Women in the Feminist Movement*. Oxford: Oxford University Press, 2006.

Breland, Lauren. "Lost Libido, or Just Forgotten? The Legal and Social Influences on Sexual Activity in Long-Term Care." *Law and Psychology Review* 38 (2014): 177–92.

Breslow, Jacob. "The Theory and Practice of Childhood: Interrogating Childhood as a Technology of Power." PhD thesis, London School of Economics and Political Science, 2016.

Bressler, Lauren, and Abraham Lavender. "Sexual Fulfillment of Heterosexual, Bisexual, and Homosexual Women." In *Historical, Literary, and Erotic Aspects of Lesbianism*, edited by Monika Kehoe, 109–22. New York: Haworth Press, 1986.

Brock, Linda J., and Glen Jennings. "Sexuality and Intimacy." In *Handbook of Gerontology: Evidence-Based Approaches to Theory, Practice, and Policy*, edited by James A. Blackburn and Catherine N. Dulmus, 244–68. Hoboken, NJ: John Wiley and Sons, 2007.

Brotto, Lori, and Morag A. Yule. "Physiological and Subjective Sexual Arousal in Self-Identified Asexual Women." *Archives of Sexual Behavior* 40, no. 4 (2011): 699–712.

Brotto, Lori and Morag Yule. "Asexuality: Sexual Orientation, Paraphilia, Sexual Dysfunction, or None of the Above?" *Archives of Sexual Behavior* 46, no. 3 (2017): 619–27.

Brown, Cole. "The Histroy of the Asexual Community." Presented at *Asexual Countercultures: Exploring Ace Communities and Intimacies,* Vancouver, BC, Simon Fraser University, November 2, 2017.

Brown, Helen Gurley. *Sex and the Single Girl: The Unmarried Woman's Guide to Men.* New York: Pocket Books, 1962.

Brown, Rita Mae. *A Plain Brown Rapper.* Oakland, CA: Diana Press, 1976.

———. *Rubyfruit Jungle.* New York: Bantam Books, 1973.

Bruhm, Steven, and Natasha Hurley. *Curiouser: On the Queerness of Children.* Minneapolis: University of Minnesota Press, 2004.

Cacchioni, Thea. "Heterosexuality and 'the Labour of Love': A Contribution to Recent Debates on Female Sexual Dysfunction." *Sexualities* 10, no. 3 (2007): 299–320.

Carland, Tammy Rae. Personal website. http://www.tammyraecarland.com/lesbianbeds.htm.

Carrigan, Mark. "There's More to Life Than Sex? Difference and Commonality within the Asexual Community." *Sexualities* 14, no. 4 (2011): 462–78.

Carter, Julian B. *The Heart of Whiteness: Normal Sexuality and Race in America, 1880–1940.* Durham, NC: Duke University Press, 2012.

Carter, Sarah. *The Importance of Being Monogamous: Marriage and Nation Building in Western Canada to 1915.* Edmonton: University of Alberta Press, 2008.

Casper, Monica J., and Lisa Jean Moore. *Missing Bodies: The Politics of Visibility.* New York: New York University Press, 2009.

Castiglia, Christopher. "Sex Panics, Sex Publics, Sex Memories." *Boundary 2* 27, no. 2 (2000): 149–75.

Castle, Terry. *The Apparitional Lesbian: Female Homosexuality and Modern Culture.* New York: Columbia University Press, 1993.

Cavanagh, Sheila L. *Sexing the Teacher: School Sex Scandals and Queer Pedagogies.* Vancouver: University of British Columbia Press, 2007.

———. "Trans* Photography, Sexual Difference and the m/Other in Vivek Shraya's *Trisha.*" Sexuality Studies Association. Toronto: Ryerson University, May 28, 2017. http://sheila.info.yorku.ca/keynotes-and-public-presentations/.

Cerankowski, KJ. "Spectacular Asexuals: Media Visibility and Cultural Fetish." In *Asexualities: Feminist and Queer Perspectives,* edited by KJ Cerankowski and M. Milks, 139–61. New York: Routledge, 2014.

Cerankowski, KJ, and M. Milks, eds. *Asexualities: Feminist and Queer Perspectives.* New York: Routledge, 2014.

Cerankowski, KJ, and M. Milks. "New Orientations: Asexuality and Its Implications for Theory and Practice." *Feminist Studies* 36, no. 3 (2010): 650–64.

Chasin, CJ DeLuzio. "Making Sense in and of the Asexual Community: Navigating Relationships and Identities in a Context of Resistance." *Journal of Community & Applied Social Psychology* 25, no. 2 (2015): 177–80.

Cholodenko, Lisa, dir. *The Kids Are All Right.* Los Angeles: Gilbert Films, 2010.

Chu, Erica. "Radical Identity Politics: Asexuality and Contemporary Articulations of Identity." In *Asexualities: Feminist and Queer Perspectives,* edited by KJ Cerankowski and M. Milks, 79–99. New York: Routledge, 2014.

Coates, Ta-Nehisi. *Between the World and Me.* New York City: Spiegel and Grau, 2015.

Cobb, Michael. *Single: Arguments for the Uncoupled.* New York: New York University Press, 2012.

Cohen, Jacqueline, and Sandra Byers. "Beyond Lesbian Bed Death: Enhancing Our Understanding of the Sexuality of Sexual-Minority Women in Relationships." *Journal of Sex Research* 51, no. 8 (2014): 893–903.

Cole, Thomas. *The Journey of Life: A Cultural History of Aging in America.* Cambridge: Cambridge University Press, 1992.

Coleman, Emily, Peter Hoon, and Emily Hoon. "Arousability and Sexual Satisfaction in Lesbian and Heterosexual Women." *Journal of Sex Research* 19, no. 1 (1983): 58–73.

Collins, Patricia Hill. *Black Feminist Thought: Knowledge, Consciousness, and the Politics of Empowerment.* New York: Routledge, 1990.

Combahee River Collective. "A Black Feminist Statement." In *All the Women Are White, All the Blacks Are Men, But Some of Us Are Brave: Black Women's Studies,* edited by Gloria T. Hull, Patricia Bell Scott, and Barbara Smith, 13–22. Old Westbury, NY: The Feminist Press, 1982.

Cooper, Brittney. *Beyond Respectability: The Intellectual Thought of Race Women.* Urbana: University of Illinois Press, 2017.

Cornelison, Laci J., and Gayle M. Doll. "Management of Sexual Expression in Long-Term Care: Ombudsmen's Perspectives." *The Gerontologist* 53, no. 5 (2012): 780–89.

Cott, Nancy F. "Passionlessness: An Interpretation of Victorian Sexual Ideology, 1790–1850." *Signs: Journal of Women in Culture and Society* 4, no. 2 (Winter 1978): 219–36.

Coviello, Peter. *Tomorrow's Parties: Sex and the Untimely in Nineteenth-Century America.* New York: New York University Press, 2013.

Cowan, Liza. "Response." *Meta Watershed,* 2010. http://maggiesmetawatershed.blogspot.ca/2010/12/sisterhood-feels-good.html.

Crawford, Margo Natalie. "Must Revolution Be a Family Affair? Revisiting *The Black Woman.*" In *Want to Start a Revolution?: Radical Women in the Black Freedom Struggle,* edited by Dayo F. Gore, Jeanne Theoharis, Komozi Woodard, 185–204. New York: New York University Press, 2009.

Crimp, Douglas. *AIDS: Cultural Analysis/Cultural Activism.* Cambridge: MIT Press, 1988.

Cryle, Peter, and Alison Moore, eds. *Frigidity: An Intellectual History.* New York: Palgrave Macmillan, 2012.

Cvetkovich, Ann. *An Archive of Feelings.* Durham, NC: Duke University Press, 2003.

Daly, Mary. *Gyn/Ecology: The Metaethics of Radical Feminism.* Boston: Beacon Press, 1978/1990.

Davis, Angela. "Racism, Birth Control, and Reproductive Rights." In *Women, Race, and Class,* 202–21. New York: Vintage Books, 1983.

De Veaux, Alexis. *Warrior Poet: A Biography of Audre Lorde.* New York: W. W. Norton, 2004.

Deacon, Susan, Victor Minichiello, and David Plummer. "Sexuality and Older People: Revisiting the Assumptions." *Educational Gerontology* 21, no. 5 (1995): 497–513.

Decker, Julie Sondra. *The Invisible Orientation: An Introduction to Asexuality.* New York: Skyhorse Publishing, 2016.

DeLamater, John, and Morgan Sill. "Sexual Desire in Later Life." *The Journal of Sex Research* 42, no. 2 (2005): 138–49.

D'Emilio, John, and Estelle B. Freedman. *Intimate Matters: A History of Sexuality in America.* New York: Harper and Row, 1988.

Densmore, Dana. "Independence from the Sexual Revolution." In *Notes from the Third Year: Women's Liberation,* 56–61. New York: New York Radical Feminists, 1971.

———. "On Celibacy." *No More Fun and Games* 1 (1968/1970): not paginated.

———. "Sexuality." *No More Fun and Games* 1 (1968/1970): not paginated.

Dickel, Simon. "Between Mumblecore and Post-Black Aesthetics: Barry Jenkins's *Medicine for Melancholy.*" In *Understanding Blackness through Performance: Contemporary Arts and the Representation of Identity,* edited by Anne Crémieux, Xavier Lemoine, and Jean-Paul Rocchi, 109–23. Basingstoke: Palgrave Macmillan, 2013.

Doan, Laura. Introduction to *Old Maids to Radical Spinsters: Unmarried Women in the Twentieth-Century Novel,* edited by Laura Doan, 1–16. Urbana: University of Illinois Press, 1991.

Douglas, Carol Anne. "Interview: Dana Densmore: Self-Defense and Feminism." *Off Our Backs* 5, no. 1 (1975): 8–9, 19.

Douglas, Carol Anne, and Alice Henry. "Towards a Politics of Sexuality." *Off Our Backs* 12, no. 6 (1982): 2–4, 20–21.

Douglas, Mary. *Purity and Danger: An Analysis of the Concepts of Pollution and Taboo.* London: Routledge and Kegan Paul, 1966.

Driskill, Qwo-Li. "Stolen from Our Bodies: First Nations Two-Spirits/Queers and the Journey to a Sovereign Erotic." *Studies in American Indian Literatures* 16, no. 2 (2004): 50–64.

Duggan, Lisa. *The Twilight of Equality.* Boston, Beacon Press, 2003.

Dunbar-Ortiz, Roxanne. "Asexuality." *No More Fun and Games* 1 (1968/1970): not paginated.

———. "Female Liberation as the Basis for Social Revolution." *No More Fun and Games* 2 (1969): 103–15.

———. "'Sexual Liberation': More of the Same Thing." *No More Fun and Games* 3 (1969): 49–56.

Echols, Alice. *Daring to Be Bad: Radical Feminism in America, 1967–1975.* Minneapolis: University of Minnesota Press, 1989.

Edmonds, Alexander. "Surgery-for-Life: Aging, Sexual Fitness and Self Management in Brazil." *Anthropology and Aging Quarterly* 34, no. 4 (2014): 246–59.

Ehrenfeld, Mally, Nili Tabak, Gila Bronner, and Rebecca Bergman. "Ethical Dilemmas Concerning the Sexuality of Elderly Patients Suffering from Dementia." *International Journal of Nursing Practice* 3, no. 4 (1997): 255–59.

Ellis, Havelock. *Studies in the Psychology of Sex: Analysis of the Sexual Impulse, Love and Pain, and the Sexual Impulse in Women.* Philadelphia: Davis, 1912.

Emens, Elizabeth F. "Compulsory Sexuality." *Stanford Law Review* 66, no. 2 (2014): 303–86.

Enck-Wanzer, Darrel, ed. *The Young Lords: A Reader.* New York: New York University Press, 2010.

Eng, David. *The Feeling of Kinship: Queer Liberalism and the Racialization of Intimacy.* Durham, NC: Duke University Press, 2010.

Enke, Finn. "Collective Memory and Transfeminist 1970s: Toward a Less Plausible History." *TSQ: Transgender Studies Quarterly* 5, no. 1 (2018): 9–29.

Ettinger, Bracha. *The Matrixial Borderspace.* Minneapolis: University of Minnesota Press, 2005.

Faderman, Lillian. *Surpassing the Love of Men: Romantic Friendship and Love between Women from the Renaissance to the Present.* New York: William Morrow, 1981.

Fahs, Breanne. *Firebrand Feminism: The Radical Lives of Ti-Grace Atkinson, Kathie Sarachild, Roxanne Dunbar-Ortiz, and Dana Densmore.* Washington, DC: University of Washington Press, 2018.

———. "The Radical Possibilities of Valerie Solanas." *Feminist Studies* 34, no. 3 (2008): 591–617.

———. "Radical Refusals: On the Anarchist Politics of Women Choosing Asexuality." *Sexualities* 13, no. 4 (2010): 445–61.

———. "Ti-Grace Atkinson and the Legacy of Radical Feminism." *Feminist Studies* 37, no. 3 (2011): 561–90.

———. *Valerie Solanas.* New York: The Feminist Press, 2014.

Fanon, Frantz. *Black Skin, White Masks.* Translated by Richard Philcox. New York: Grove Press, 1952/2008.

Feinberg, Leslie. *Stone Butch Blues.* Ithaca, NY: Firebrand Books, 1993.

———. "Street Transvestite Action Revolutionaries." *Workers World,* 2006. http://www.workers.org/2006/us/lavender-red-73/.

The Feminists. "Dangers in the Pro-Women Line." New York: The Feminists, mimeograph, n.d.

———. "The Feminists: A Political Organization to Annihilate Sex Roles." In *Notes from the Second Year: Women's Liberation,* edited by Shulamith Firestone and Anne Koedt, 114–18. New York: New York Radical Feminists, 1970.

Fernández, Johanna. "Denise Oliver and the Young Lords Party: Stretching the Political Boundaries of Struggle." In *Want to Start a Revolution?: Radical Women in the Black Freedom Struggle,* edited by Dayo F. Gore, Jeanne Theoharis, and Komozi Woodard, 271–93. New York: New York University Press, 2009.

Fields, Jessica. "'Children Having Children': Race, Innocence, and Sexuality Education." *Social Problems* 52, no. 4 (2005): 549–71.

Fisher, Simon D. Elin, Rasheedah Phillips, and Ido H. Katri. "Trans Temporalities (Introduction to Special Issue)." *Somatechnics* 7, no. 1 (2017): 1–15.

Foglia, Mary Beth, and Karen I. Fredriksen-Goldsen. "Health Disparities among LGBT Older Adults and the Role of Nonconscious Bias." *LGBT Bioethics: Visibility, Disparities, and Dialogue,* special report, *Hastings Center Report* 44, no. 5 (2014): S40–S44.

"Forbidden Discourse: The Silencing of Feminist Criticism of 'Gender.'" *Fire in My Belly: A Radical Feminist Blog.* 2013. https://feministuk.wordpress.com/2013/08/19/forbidden-discourse-the-silencing-of-feminist-criticism-of-gender/

Foucault, Michel. *The History of Sexuality: An Introduction, Vol. I.* Translated by Robert Hurley. New York: Vintage Books, 1978/1990.

———. "Lecture Eleven: 17 March 1976." In *Society Must Be Defended: Lectures at the College de France, 1975–1976,* 239–63. New York: Picador, 2003.

Fraiman, Susan. *Cool Men and the Second Sex.* New York: Columbia University Press, 2003.

Franzen, Trisha. *Spinsters and Lesbians: Independent Womanhood in the United States.* New York: New York University Press, 1996.

Fraser, Nancy. "Rethinking the Public Sphere: A Contribution to the Critique of Actually Existing Democracy." *Social Text* 25, no. 26 (1990): 56–80.

Freccero, Carla. *Queer/Early/Modern.* Durham, NC: Duke University Press, 2006.

Freeman, Elizabeth. *Time Binds: Queer Temporalities, Queer Histories.* Durham, NC: Duke University Press, 2010.

Freud, Sigmund. *Civilization and Its Discontents.* Translated by James Strachey. New York: Norton, 1930/1961.

———. "Female Sexuality." In *Standard Edition of the Complete Psychological Works V. 21 (1927–1931),* translated by James Strachey, 225–43. London: Hogarth Press, 1961.

———. *Introductory Lectures on Psychoanalysis.* Translated by James Strachey. Penguin Freud Library Volume 1. London: Penguin, 1973.

———. *Three Essays on the Theory of Sexuality.* Translated by James Strachey. New York: Basic Books, 1905/1975.

———. *The "Wolf" Man.* Translated by Louise Adey Huish. London, Penguin Books, 1918/2002.

Friedan, Betty. *It Changed My Life: Writings on the Women's Movement.* New York: Random House, 1976.

Froide, Amy. *Never Married: Singlewomen in Early Modern England.* Oxford: Oxford University Press, 2005.

Frye, Marilyn. "Lesbian 'Sex.'" In *Willful Virgin: Essays in Feminism, 1976–1992,* 109–19. Freedom, CA: Crossing Press, 1992.

Gallop, Jane. "Observations of a Mother." In *The Familial Gaze,* edited by Marianne Hirsch, 67–84. Hanover, NH: Dartmouth College, 1999.

Gavey, Nicola. *Just Sex? The Cultural Scaffolding of Rape.* London: Routledge, 2005.

Gerhard, Jane. *Desiring Revolution: Second Wave Feminism and the Rewriting of American Sexual Thought, 1920 to 1982.* New York: Columbia University Press, 2001.

Gilmore, Ruth Wilson. *Golden Gulag: Prisons, Surplus, Crisis, and Opposition in Globalizing California.* Berkeley: University of California Press, 2007.

Ginoza, Mary Kame, Tristan Miller, and the AVEN Survey Team. *The 2014 AVEN Community Census: Preliminary Findings.* 2014. https://asexualcensus.files.wordpress.com /2014/11/2014censuspreliminaryreport.pdf.

Giroux, Henry. *Stealing Innocence: Youth, Corporate Power, and the Politics of Culture.* New York: St. Martin's Press, 2000.

Goffman, Erving. *Asylums: Essays on the Social Situation of Mental Patients and Other Inmates.* Garden City, NY: Anchor Books, 1961.

Gore, Dayo F., Jeanne Theoharis, and Komozi Woodard, eds. *Want to Start a Revolution?: Radical Women in the Black Freedom Struggle.* New York: New York University Press, 2009.

Gott, Marryn. *Sexuality, Sexual Health and Ageing.* Berkshire: Open University Press, 2005.

Gott, Merryn, and Sharron Hinchliff. "How Important Is Sex in Later Life? The Views of Older People." *Social Science and Medicine* 56, no. 8 (2003): 1617–28.

Gottschalk, Donna. "SISTERHOOD FEELS GOOD." Times Change Press, 1971 (photograph 1969).

Grace, Sebastian. "What's R(ace) and RAD Got to Do with It? Musings of a Transracially Adopted Asexual." In *Brown and Gray,* edited by jnramos, 2015.

Griffin, Farah Jasmine. "Conflict and Chorus: Reconsidering Toni Cade's *The Black Woman: An Anthology.*" In *Is It Nation Time?: Contemporary Essays on Black Power and Black Nationalism,* edited by Eddie S. Glaude, 113–29. Chicago: University of Chicago Press, 2002.

Gupta, Kristina. "Asexuality and Disability: Mutual Negation in *Adams v. Rice* and New Directions for Coalition Building." In *Asexualities: Feminist and Queer Perspectives,* edited by KJ Cerankowski and M. Milks, 283–301. New York: Routledge, 2014.

———. "Compulsory Sexuality: Evaluating an Emerging Concept." *Signs: Journal of Women in Culture and Society* 41, no. 1 (2015): 131–54.

———. "Picturing Space for Lesbian Nonsexualities: Rethinking Sex-Normative Commitments through *The Kids Are All Right* (2010)." *Journal of Lesbian Studies* 17, no. 1 (2013): 103–18.

———. "'Screw Health': Representations of Sex as a Health-Promoting Activity in Medical and Popular Literature." *Journal of Medical Humanities* 32, no. 2 (2011): 127–40.

Gupta, Kristina, and Thea Cacchioni. "Sexual Improvement as if Your Health Depends on It: An Analysis of Contemporary Sex Manuals." *Feminism & Psychology* 23, no. 4 (2013): 442–58.

Gupta, Kristina, and KJ Cerankowski. "Asexualities and Media." In *The Routledge Companion to Media, Sex, and Sexuality,* edited by Clarissa Smith, Feona Attwood, and Brian McNair, 19–26. New York: Routledge, 2018.

Halberstam, Jack. *In a Queer Time and Place.* New York: New York University Press, 2005.

———. "The Kids Aren't Alright!" *Bully Bloggers,* July 15, 2010. http://bullybloggers.wordpress.com/2010/07/15/the-kids-arent-alright/.

———. *The Queer Art of Failure.* Durham, NC: Duke University Press, 2011.

Hammond, Harmony. *Lesbian Art in America: A Contemporary History.* New York: Rizzoli, 2000.

Hastings, Donald W. *Impotence and Frigidity.* Boston: Little, Brown, 1963.

"The Haven for the Human Amoeba." *Yahoo Groups.* http://groups.yahoo.com/group/havenforthehumanamoeba/.

Hawkins Owen, Ianna. "Asexuality, Incarceration, and Black Power(lessness)." Presented November 18, 2017, at the National Women's Studies Association annual conference, Baltimore, MD.

———. "On the Racialization of Asexuality." In *Asexualities: Feminist and Queer Perspectives,* edited by KJ Cerankowski and M. Milks, 119–35. New York: Routledge, 2014.

———. "Still, Nothing: Mammy and Black Asexual Possibility," *Feminist Review* 120, no. 1 (2018): 70–84.

Hedblom, Jack. "Dimensions of Lesbian Sexual Experience." *Archives of Sexual Behavior* 2, no. 4 (1973): 329–41.

Hesford, Victoria. "Feminism and Its Ghosts: The Spectre of the Feminist-as-Lesbian." *Feminist Theory* 6, no. 3 (2005): 227–50.

Hill, Bridget. *Women Alone: Spinsters in England 1660–1850.* New Haven, CT: Yale University Press, 2001.

Hill Collins, Patricia. "Toward a New Vision: Race, Class, and Gender as Categories of Analysis and Connection." *Race, Sex & Class* 1, no. 1 (1993): 25–45.

Hills, Rachel. *The Sex Myth.* New York: Simon and Schuster, 2015.

Hinchliff, Sharon, and Marryn Gott. "Challenging Social Myths and Stereotypes of Women and Aging: Heterosexual Women Talk about Sex." *Journal of Women and Aging* 20, no. 1/2 (2008): 65–81.

Hinderliter, Andrew. *Asexuality: The History of a Definition | Asexual Explorations.* 2009. http://www.asexualexplorations.net/home/history_of_definition.html.

Hogeland, Lisa Maria. "Sexuality in the Consciousness-Raising Novel of the 1970s." *Journal of the History of Sexuality* 5, no. 4 (1995): 601–32.

Holland, Sharon Patricia. *The Erotic Life of Racism*. Durham, NC: Duke University Press, 2012.

Hollway, Wendy. "Gender Difference and the Production of Subjectivity (1984)." In *Changing the Subject: Psychology, Social Regulation and Subjectivity*, 227–263. London: Routledge, 1998.

Holmes, David, Jacob Reingold, and Jeanne Teresi. "Sexual Expression and Dementia. Views of Caregivers: A Pilot Study." *International Journal of Geriatric Psychiatry* 12, no. 7 (1997): 696–701.

hooks, bell. "Are You Still A Slave? Liberating the Black Female Body." New York: The New School, 2014.

———. "The Oppositional Gaze: Black Female Spectators." In *Black Looks: Race and Representation*, 115–31. Boston: South End Press, 1992.

Hopkins, Pauline. "Higher Education of Colored Women in White Schools and Colleges (1902)." In *Daughter of the Revolution*, edited by Ira Dworkin, 193–98. New Brunswick, NJ: Rutgers University Press, 2007.

*House* (television series). Los Angeles: Fox Network, 2012.

Huffer, Lynne. *Are the Lips a Grave? A Queer Feminist on the Ethics of Sex*. New York: Columbia University Press, 2013.

Huyck, Margaret Hellie. "Romantic Relationship in Later Life." *Generations* 25, no. 2 (2001): 9–17.

Iasenza, Suzanne. "Lesbian Sexuality Post-Stonewall to Post-Modernism: Putting the 'Lesbian Bed Death' Concept to Bed." *Journal of Sex Education and Therapy* 25, no. 1 (2000): 59–69.

Irvine, Janice, M. *Disorders of Desire: Sexuality and Gender in Modern American Sexology*. Philadelphia: Temple University Press, 1990/2005.

"'It's Not a Viewing Platform, It's an Experience': Tracey Emin Prepares to Put Bed on View at Tate Britain." *Culture24*, March 20, 2015. http://www.culture24.org.uk/art/art522146-not-a-viewing-platform-an-experience-tracey-emin-prepares-to-put-bed-on-view-at-tate-britain.

Jagose, Annamarie. "Counterfeit Pleasures: Fake Orgasm and Queer Agency." *Textual Practice* 24, no. 3 (2010): 517–39.

———. *Orgasmology*. Durham, NC: Duke University Press, 2013.

Jay, David. *A Look at Online Collective Identity Formation*. May 13, 2003.

Jnramos, ed. *Brown and Gray* (2015): 36 pages.

Jochild, Maggie. "SISTERHOOD FEELS GOOD." *Meta Watershed*, 2010. http://maggiesmetawatershed.blogspot.ca/2010/12/sisterhood-feels-good.html.

Johnson, Anne M., Jane Wadsworth, Kaye Wellings, Julia Field, and Sally Bradshaw. *Sexual Attitudes and Lifestyles*. London: Blackwell Scientific Publications, 1994.

Johnson, Myra T. "Asexual and Autoerotic Women: Two Invisible Groups." In *The Sexually Oppressed*, edited by Harvey L. Gochros and Jean S. Gochros, 96–109. New York: Association Press, 1977.

Kafer, Alison. *Feminist, Queer, Crip*. Bloomington: Indiana University Press, 2013.

Kahan, Benjamin. *Celibacies: American Modernism and Sexual Life*. Durham, NC: Duke University Press, 2013.

Katz, Jonathan. "The Art of Code." In *Significant Others*, edited by Whotney Chadwick and Isabelle de Courtivron, 189–208. New York: Thames and Hudson, 1993. http://www.queer-arts.org/archive/show4/forum/katz/katz_set.html.

Katz, Stephen. "Hold On! Falling, Embodiment, and the Materiality of Old Age." In *Corpus,* edited by Monica J. Casper and Paisley Currah, 187–205. New York: Palgrave Macmillan, 2011.

Katz, Stephen, and Barbara Marshall. "Forever Functional: Sexual Fitness and the Ageing Male Body." *Body & Society* 8, no. 4 (2002): 43–70.

———. "New Sex for Old: Lifestyle, Consumerism, and the Ethics of Aging Well." *Journal of Aging Studies* 17, no. 1 (2003): 3–16.

Katz, Sue. "Smash Phallic Imperialism" (sometimes printed as "The Sensuous Woman"). In *Out of the Closets: Voices of Gay Liberation,* edited by Karla Jay and Allen Young, 259–62. New York: New York University Press, 1971/1992.

Kelley, Robin. *Freedom Dreams: The Black Radical Imagination.* Boston: Beacon Press, 2002.

Kelly, Casey Ryan. "Elliot Rodger's Retribution: The Thanatopolitics of Involuntary Celibacy." Forthcoming.

Kent, Kathryn. *Making Girls into Women: American Women's Writing.* Durham, NC: Duke University Press, 2003.

Khanna, Ranjana. "Disposability." *differences: A Journal of Feminist Cultural Studies* 20, no. 1 (2009): 181–98.

Kim, Eunjung. "Asexualities and Disabilities in Constructing Sexual Normalcy." In *Asexualities: Feminist and Queer Perspectives,* edited by KJ Cerankowski and M. Milks, 249–82. New York: Routledge, 2014.

———. "Asexuality in Disability Narratives." *Sexualities* 14, no. 4 (2011): 479–93.

———. "How Much Sex Is Healthy? The Pleasures of Asexuality." In *Against Health: How Health Became the New Morality,* edited by Jonathan M. Metzl and Anna Kirkland, 157–69. New York: New York University Press, 2010.

Kincaid, James. *Erotic Innocence.* Durham, NC: Duke University Press, 1998.

Kinsey, Alfred C., Wardell B. Pomeroy, and Clyde E. Martin. *Sexual Behavior in the Human Male.* Philadelphia: W. B. Saunders, 1948.

Kinsey, Alfred C., Wardell B. Pomeroy, Clyde E. Martin, and Paul H. Gebhard. *Sexual Behavior in the Human Female.* Philadelphia: W. B. Saunders, 1953.

Koedt, Anne. "The Myth of the Vaginal Orgasm." In *Notes from the Second Year: Women's Liberation,* 37–41. New York: New York Radical Feminists, 1968/1970.

Kohan, Jenji, prod. *Orange Is the New Black* (television series). Santa Monica: Lionsgate Television, 2013.

Krafft-Ebing, Richard von. *Psychopathia Sexualis with Especial Reference to Contrary Sexual Instincts: A Clinical Forensic Study.* 12th ed. Translated by Charles G. Chaddock. New York: Rebman, 1886/1922.

Kranidis, Rita. *The Victorian Spinster and Colonial Emigration: Contested Subjects.* New York: St. Martin's Press, 1999.

Krestan, Jo-Ann, and Claudia Bepko. "The Problem of Fusion in the Lesbian Relationship." *Family Process* 19, no. 3 (1980): 277–89.

Kristeva, Julia. *The Powers of Horror: An Essay on Abjection.* Translated by Leon S. Roudiez. New York: Columbia University Press, 1982.

Lacan, Jacques. "The Split between the Eye and the Gaze." In *The Four Fundamental Concepts of Psychoanalysis. The Seminar of Jacques Lacan,* Book 11. Translated by Alan Sheridan. London: W. W. Norton, 1981.

Lakshmi Piepzna-Samarasinha, Leah. *Bodymap: Poems.* Toronto: Mawenzi House, 2015.

Lasky, Kyle. Personal website. http://www.kylelasky.com/lesbian-bedrooms-ii.

Lee, Spike. *Chi-Raq.* Santa Monica: Amazon Studios, 2015.

Lesnik-Oberstein, Karín. "Childhood, Queer Theory, and Feminism." *Feminist Theory* 11, no. 3 (2010): 309–21.

Lewis, Brigitte. "The Era of Lesbian Bed Death Is Over, Long Live Lesbian Fuck Eye." *Archer Magazine,* September 9, 2015. http://archermagazine.com.au/2015/09/the-era-of-lesbian-bed-death-is-over-long-live-lesbian-fuck-eye/.

Lief, Harold. "What's New in Sexual Research? Inhibited Sexual Desire." *Medical Aspects of Human Sexuality* 11 (1977): 94–95.

Lightfoot, Elizabeth. "Disability." In *Handbook of Gerontology: Evidence-Based Approaches to Theory, Practice, and Policy,* edited by James A. Blackburn and Catherine N. Dulmus, 201–29. Hoboken, NJ: John Wiley and Sons, 2007.

Lindemann Nelson, Hilde. "Stories of My Old Age." In *Mother Time: Women, Aging, Ethics,* edited by Margaret Urban Walker, 75–95. New York: Rowman and Littlefield, 2000.

Lipschutz, Barbara. "Nobody Needs to Get Fucked." *Lesbian Voices* 1, no. 4 (1975): 57.

Loe, Meika. "Sex and the Senior Woman: Pleasure and Danger in the Viagra Era." *Sexualities* 7, no. 3 (2004): 303–26.

Lorde, Audre. "Scratching the Surface: Some Notes on Barriers to Women and Loving" (1978). In *Sister Outsider,* 45–52. Freedom, CA: The Crossing Press, 1984.

———. "Sexism: An American Disease in Blackface" (1979). In *Sister Outsider,* 60–65. Freedom, CA: The Crossing Press, 1984.

———. "Uses of the Erotic: The Erotic as Power" (1978). In *Sister Outsider,* 53–59. Freedom, CA: The Crossing Press, 1984.

Lorde, Audre, and Adrienne Rich. "An Interview: Audre Lorde and Adrienne Rich" (1979). In *Sister Outsider,* 81–109. Freedom, CA: The Crossing Press, 1984.

Love, Heather. "Compulsory Happiness and Queer Existence." *New Formations: A Journal of Culture/Theory/Politics* 63 (2007): 52–64.

———. *Feeling Backward: Loss and the Politics of Queer History.* Cambridge, MA: Harvard University Press, 2007.

———. "Gyn/Apology: Sarah Orne Jewett's Spinster Aesthetics." *ESQ: A Journal of American Renaissance* 55, no. 3–4 (2009): 305–34.

Luciano, Dana. *Arranging Grief: Sacred Time and the Body in Nineteenth-Century.* New York: New York University Press, 2007.

Luna, Caleb. "Romantic Love Is Killing Us: Who Takes Care of Us When We Are Single?" *The Body Is Not An Apology,* 2016. https://thebodyisnotanapology.com/magazine/romantic-love-is-killing-us/.

Lund, Emily, and Bayley Johnson. "Asexuality and Disability: Strange but Compatible Bedfellows." *Sexuality and Disability* 33, no. 1 (2015): 123–32.

MacInnis, Cara C., and Gordon Hodson. "'Intergroup Bias towards "Group X': Evidence of Prejudice, Dehumanization, Avoidance, and Discrimination against Asexuals." *Group Processes and Intergroup Relations* 15, no. 6 (2012): 725–43.

MacNeela, Pádraig, and Aisling Murphy. "Freedom, Invisibility, and Community: A Qualitative Study of Self-Identification with Asexuality." *Archives of Sexual Behavior* 44, no. 3 (2015): 799–812.

Maisha. *Taking the Cake: An Illustrated Primer on Asexuality* (2012): 12 pages.

Masters, William, and Virginia Johnson. *Homosexuality in Perspective*. Boston: Little, Brown, 1979.

———. *Human Sexual Response*. New York: Bantam Books, 1966.

Masters, William H., Virginia E. Johnson, and Robert C. Kolodny. *Masters and Johnson on Sex and Human Loving*. Boston: Little, Brown, 1986.

Mawhinney, Janet Lee. "'Giving up the Ghost': Disrupting the (Re)production of White Privilege in Anti-racist Pedagogy and Organizational Change." Master's thesis, Ontario Institute for Studies in Education of the University of Toronto, 1998.

Maynard, Robyn. *Policing Black Lives: State Violence in Canada from Slavery to the Present*. Black Point: Fernwood Publishing, 2017.

Mbembe, Achille. "Necropolitics." *Public Culture* 15, no. 1 (2003): 11–40.

McGlotten, Shaka, and Lisa Jean Moore. "The Geriatric Clinic: Dry and Limp: Aging Queers, Zombies, and Sexual Reanimation." *Journal of Medical Humanities* 34, no. 2 (2013): 261–68.

McGregor, Hannah. "The Loneliness of the Spinster." *Chronicle Vitae*, 2016. https://chroniclevitae.com/news/1609-the-loneliness-of-the-spinster.

Meagher, Michelle. "Jenny Saville and a Feminist Aesthetics of Disgust." *Hypatia* 18, no. 4 (2003): 23–41.

Metzl, Jonathan M., and Anna Kirkland, eds. *Against Health: How Health Became the New Morality*. New York: New York University Press, 2010.

Milks, M. "Stunted Growth: Asexual Politics and the Rhetoric of Sexual Liberation." In *Asexualities: Feminist and Queer Perspectives*, edited by KJ Cerankowski and M. Milks, 100–118. New York: Routledge, 2014.

Miller-Young, Mireille. *A Taste for Brown Sugar: Black Women in Pornography*. Durham, NC: Duke University Press, 2014.

Mills, Charles W. *The Racial Contract*. Ithaca, NY: Cornell University Press, 1997.

Minichiello, Victor, David Plummer, and Anne Seal. "The 'Asexual' Older Person? Australian Evidence." *Venereology* 9, no. 3 (1996): 180–88.

Minkler, Meredith, and Pamela Fadem. "'Successful Aging': A Disability Perspective." *Journal of Disability Policy Studies* 12, no. 4 (2002): 229–35.

Mondé, Geniece Crawford. "#BlackDontCrack: A Content Analysis of the Aging Black Woman in Social Media." *Feminist Media Studies* 18, no. 1 (2018): 47–60.

Morales, Iris. "¡Palante, Siempre Palante! The Young Lords." In *The Puerto Rican Movement: Voices from the Diaspora*, edited by Andrés Torres and José E. Velázquez, 210–27. Philadelphia: Temple University Press, 1998.

Morgan, Robin, ed. *Sisterhood Is Powerful: An Anthology of Writings from the Women's Liberation Movement*. New York: Random House, 1970.

Morrigan, Clementine. "Trauma Time: The Queer Temporalities of the Traumatized Mind." *Somatechnics* 7, no. 1 (2017): 50–58.

Morrissey, A. K. "Remedial Asexuality: Sexualnormativity in Health Care." In *The Remedy: Queer and Trans Voices on Health and Health Care*, edited by Zena Sherman, 165–83. Vancouver: Arsenal Pulp Press, 2016.

Moynihan, Daniel Patrick. *The Negro Family: The Case for National Action.* Washington, DC: GPO, 1965.

Muñoz, José Esteban. *Cruising Utopia: The Then and There of Queer Futurity.* New York: New York University Press, 2009.

———. "Feeling Brown: Ethnicity and Affect in Ricardo Bracho's *The Sweetest Hangover (and Other STDs)*." *Theatre Journal* 52, no. 1 (2000): 67–79.

Muehlbauer, Melissa, and Patricia Crane. "Elder Abuse and Neglect." *Journal of Psychosocial Nursing and Mental Health Services* 44, no. 11 (2006): 43–48.

Nair, Yasmin. "Your Sex Is Not Radical." June 7, 2015. http://yasminnair.net/content/your-sex-not-radical.

Negrin, Sue. "A Weekend in Lesbian Nation." *It Ain't Me, Babe* 2, no. 1 (1971): 11.

Nelson, Jennifer. *Women of Color and the Reproductive Rights Movement.* New York: New York University Press, 2003.

Nelson, Maggie. *The Argonauts.* Minneapolis, MN: Graywolf Press, 2015.

Neugerbauer-Visano, Robynne, ed. *Seniors and Sexuality: Experiencing Intimacy in Later Life.* Toronto: Canadian Scholars' Press, 1998.

Newmahr, Staci. "Eroticism as Embodied Emotion: The Erotics of Renaissance Faire." *Symbolic Interaction* 37, no. 2 (2014): 209–25.

Nichols, Margaret. "The Treatment of Inhibited Sexual Desire (ISD) in Lesbian Couples." *Women & Therapy* 1, no. 4 (1982): 49–66.

Nurius, Paula S. "Mental Health Implications of Sexual Orientation." *The Journal of Sex Research* 19, no. 2 (1983): 119–36.

O'Donnell, Ellen. "Thoughts on Celibacy." *No More Fun and Games* 1 (1968/1970): not paginated.

Oliver, Denise. "We Were Young Lords, Not Young Ladies." *Daily Kos.* August 22, 2009. https://www.dailykos.com/stories/2009/8/22/770157/—.

O'Mara, Michele. "The Correlation of Sexual Frequency and Relationship Satisfaction among Lesbians." PhD diss., American Academy of Clinical Sexologists, Florida, 2012.

Opie, Catherine. *Self-Portrait/Cutting.* 1993. Guggenheim Museum, New York. https://artsandculture.google.com/asset/self-portrait-cutting/yQG2x2FpePzJXw.

———. *Self-Portrait/Nursing.* 2004. Guggenheim Museum, New York. https://artsandculture.google.com/asset/self-portrait-nursing/SgH0N6WN0_B8gw.

O'Reilly, Zoe. "My Life as an Amoeba." *StarNet Dispatches*, 1997.

Oudshoorn, Nelly. *Beyond the Natural Body: An Archaeology of Sex Hormones.* New York: Routledge, 1994.

Paige, Peter, et al., prod. *The Fosters* (television series). Burbank: ABC Family, 2013.

Patton, Gwen. "Black People and the Victorian Ethos." In *The Black Woman: An Anthology*, edited by Toni Cade Bambara, 143–48. New York: New American Library, 1970.

Persson, Tove, and David Wästerfors. "'Such Trivial Matters': How Staff Account for Restrictions of Residents' Influence in Nursing Homes." *Journal of Aging Studies* 23, no. 1 (2009): 1–11.

Phillips, Joy, and Genée Marks. "Ageing Lesbians: Marginalizing Discourses and Social Exclusion in the Aged Care Industry." *Journal of Lesbian and Gay Social Services* 20, no. 1/2 (2008): 187–202.

Phillips, Linda R., Guifang Guo, and Haesook Kim. "Elder Mistreatment in U. S. Residential Care Facilities: The Scope of the Problem." *Journal of Elder Abuse & Neglect* 25, no. 1 (2013): 19–39.

Pines, Davida. *The Marriage Paradox: Modernist Novels and the Cultural Imperative to Marry.* Gainesville: University of Florida Press, 2006.

Plato. *Symposium.* Translated by C. J. Rowe. Warminster: Aris and Phillips, 1998.

Pleschberger, Sabine. "Dignity and the Challenge of Dying in Nursing Homes: The Residents' View." *Age and Ageing* 36, no. 2 (2007): 197–202.

Pollard, Nettie. "The Small Matter of Children." In *Bad Girls and Dirty Pictures: The Challenge to Reclaim Feminism,* edited by Alison Assiter and Avedon Carol, 105–11. London: Pluto, 1993.

Poston, Dudley L., Jr., and Amanda K. Baumle. "Patterns of Asexuality in the United States." *Demographic Research* 23 (2010): 509–30.

Potts, Annie. *The Science/Fiction of Sex: Feminist Deconstruction and the Vocabularies of Heterosex.* London: Routledge, 2002.

Potts, Annie, Nicola Gavey, Victoria M. Grace, and Tiina Vares. "The Downside of Viagra: Women's Experiences and Concerns." *Sociology of Health & Illness* 25, no. 1 (2003): 697–719.

Prause, Nicole, and Cynthia Graham. "Asexuality: Classification and Characterization." *Archives of Sexual Behavior* 36, no. 3 (2007): 341–56.

Przybylo, Ela. "Crisis and Safety: The Asexual in Sexusociety." *Sexualities* 14, no. 4 (2011): 444–61.

———. "Masculine Doubt and Sexual Wonder: Asexually-Identified Men Talk about their (A) sexualities." In *Asexualities: Feminist and Queer Perspectives,* edited by KJ Cerankowski and M. Milks, 225–46. New York: Routledge, 2014.

———. "Producing Facts: Empirical Asexuality and the Scientific Study of Sex." *Feminism & Psychology* 23, no. 2 (2013): 224–42.

Przybylo, Ela, and Danielle Cooper. "Asexual Resonances: Tracing a Queerly Asexual Archive." *GLQ: A Journal of Lesbian and Gay Studies* 20, no. 3 (2014): 297–318.

Przybylo, Ela, and Polina Ivleva. "Teaching It Straight: Sexuality Education across Post-State-Socialist Contexts." In *Childhood and Schooling in (Post)Socialist Societies: Memories of Everyday Life,* edited by Iveta Silova, Nelli Piattoeva, and Zsuzsa Millei, 183–203. London: Palgrave Macmillan, 2018.

Puar, Jasbir. *Terrorist Assemblages: Homonationalism in Queer Times.* Durham, NC: Duke University Press, 2007.

Pyne, Jake. "Arresting Ashley X: Trans Youth, Puberty Blockers and the Question of Whether Time Is on Your Side." *Somatechnics* 7, no. 1 (2017): 95–123.

Radicalesbians. "The Woman Identified Woman." In *Notes from the Third Year: Women's Liberation,* 81–84. New York: New York Radical Feminists, 1970/1971.

Randolph, Sherie M. *Florynce "Flo" Kennedy: The Life of a Black Feminist Radical.* Chapel Hill: University of North Carolina Press, 2015.

———. "'Women's Liberation or . . . Black Liberation, You're Fighting the Same Enemies': Flo-rynce Kennedy, Black Power, and Feminism." In *Want to Start a Revolution?: Radical Women in the Black Freedom Struggle,* edited by Dayo F. Gore, Jeanne Theoharis, and Komozi Woodard, 223–47. New York: New York University Press, 2009.

Ramos, Yessica. "Brown Femme and Ace." In *Brown and Gray,* edited by jnramos, 2015.

Rebec, Doroteja, Igor Karnjuš, Sabina Ličen, and Katarina Babnik. "Breaking Down Taboos Concerning Sexuality among the Elderly." In *Sexology in Midwifery,* edited by Ana Polona Mivsek, 189–207. Rijeka: InTech Open, 2015.

Rennie, Susan, and Kirsten Grimstad. *The New Woman's Survival Catalogue.* New York: Coward, McCann and Geoghegan, 1973.

Renninger, Bryce J. "'Where I Can Be Myself . . . Where I Can Speak My Mind': Networked Counterpublics in a Polymedia Environment." *New Media and Society* 17, no. 9 (2015): 1513–29.

Reynolds, Evelyn. "In America, Aging while Black Takes Solidarity, Activism and Magic." *Huffpost,* 2017. https://www.huffingtonpost.com/entry/aging-while-black-activism_us _58a477efe4b094a129f106eb.

Rich, Adrienne. "Compulsory Heterosexuality and Lesbian Existence." *Signs: Journal of Women in Culture and Society* 5, no. 4 (1980): 631–60.

Rifkin, Mark. "The Erotics of Sovereignty." In *Queer Indigenous Studies: Critical Interventions in Theory, Politics, and Literature,* edited by Qwo-Li Driskill, Chris Finley, Brian Joseph Gilley, and Scott Lauria Morgensen, 172–89. Tucson: University of Arizona Press, 2011.

———. *The Erotics of Sovereignty: Queer Native Writing in the Era of Self-Determination.* Minne-apolis: University of Minnesota Press, 2012.

———. *When Did Indians Become Straight? Kinship, the History of Sexuality, and Native Sover-eignty.* New York: Oxford University Press, 2011.

Roberts, Dorothy E. *Killing the Black Body: Race, Reproduction, and the Meaning of Liberty.* New York: Pantheon Books, 1997.

Rodger, Elliot. "My Twisted World: The Story of Elliot Rodger." 2014. https://www.document-cloud.org/documents/1173808-elliot-rodger-manifesto.html.

Rohy, Valerie. *Anachronism and Its Others: Sexuality, Race, Temporality.* New York: SUNY Press, 2009.

Rothblum, Esther D. "Early Memories, Current Realities." In *Boston Marriages: Romantic but Asexual Relationships among Contemporary Lesbians,* edited by Esther D. Rothblum and Kathleen A. Brehony, 14–18. Amherst: University of Massachusetts Press, 1993.

Rothblum, Esther, and Kathleen Brehony, eds. *Boston Marriages: Romantic but Asexual Relation-ships among Contemporary Lesbians.* Amherst: University of Massachusetts Press, 1993.

Rowe, John, and Robert Kahn. "Successful Aging." *The Gerontologist* 37, no. 4 (1997): 433–40.

Rubin, Gayle. "Thinking Sex: Notes for a Radical Theory of the Politics of Sexuality." In *Pleasure and Danger: Exploring Female Sexuality,* edited by Carole S. Vance, 267–319. London: Rout-ledge and Kegan Paul, 1984.

Samuels, Ellen. "Cripping Anti-Futurity, or, If You Love Queer Theory So Much, Why Don't You Marry It?" Annual Meeting of Society for Disability Studies. San Jose, CA, June 15–18, 2011.

Sandford, Stella. "Sexually Ambiguous." *Angelaki* 11, no. 3 (2006): 43–59.

Scherrer, Kristin. "Coming to an Asexual Identity: Negotiating Identity, Negotiating Desire." *Sexualities* 11, no. 5 (2008): 621–41.

———. "Images of Sexuality and Aging in Gerontological Literature." *Sexuality Research and Social Policy* 6, no. 4 (2009): 5–12.

Scott, Susie, and Matt Dawson. "Rethinking Asexuality: A Symbolic Interactionist Account," *Sexualities* 18, no. 1–2 (2015): 3–19.

Sears-Roberts Alterovits, Sheyna, and Gerald A. Mendelsohn. "Partner Preferences across the Life Span: Online Dating by Older Adults." *Psychology and Aging* 24, no. 2 (2009): 513–17.

Sedgwick, Eve Kosofsky. *Epistemology of the Closet.* Berkeley: University of California Press, 1990.

———. *Tendencies.* Durham, NC: Duke University Press, 1993.

Segal, Judy. "The Sexualization of the Medical." *Journal of Sex Research* 49, no. 4 (2012): 369–78.

Segal, Lynne. *Out of Time: The Pleasures and Perils of Aging.* London: Verso, 2014.

Seidman, Steven. *Romantic Longings: Love in America, 1830–1980.* New York: Routledge, 1991.

Seitler, Dana. "Making Sexuality Sensible: Tammy Rae Carland's and Catherine Opie's Queer Aesthetic Forms." In *Feeling Photography,* edited by Elspeth H. Brown and Thy Phu, 47–70. Durham, NC: Duke University Press, 2014.

Sellerberg, Ann-Mari. "Expressivity within a Time Schedule: Subordinated Interaction on Geriatric Wards." *Sociology of Health and Illness* 13, no. 1 (1991): 68–82.

Shraya, Vivek. *Trisha.* 2016. https://vivekshraya.com/visual/trisha/.

Shuttleworth, Russell. "Bridging Theory and Experience: A Critical-Interpretive Ethnography of Sexuality and Disability." In *Sex and Disability,* edited by Robert McRuer and Anna Mollow, 54–68. Durham, NC: Duke University Press, 2012.

Sichtermann, Barbara. "The Lost Eroticism of the Breasts." In *Femininity: The Politics of the Personal,* translated by John Whitlam, 55–66. Minneapolis: University of Minnesota Press, 1986.

Silver, Kenneth. "Master Bedrooms, Master Narratives: Home, Homosexuality, and Post-War Art." In *Not at Home: The Suppression of Domesticity in Modern Art and Architecture,* edited by Christopher Reed, 206–22. London: Thames and Hudson, 1996.

Simpson, Paul, Maria Horne, Laura J. E. Brown, Christine Brown Wilson, Tommy Dickinson, and Kate Torkington. "Old(er) Care Home Residents and Sexual/Intimate Citizenship." *Ageing and Society* 37, no. 2 (2016): 1–23.

Siverskog, Anna. "Ageing Bodies That Matter: Age, Gender and Embodiment in Older Transgender People's Life Stories." *NORA: Nordic Journal of Feminist and Gender Research* 23, no. 1 (2015): 4–19.

Sloan, Lorca Jolene. "Ace of (BDSM) Clubs: Building Asexual Relationships through BDSM Practice." *Sexualities* 18, no. 5 (2015): 548–63.

Smith, Barbara. "Toward a Black Feminist Criticism." (1977). *Women's Studies International Quarterly* 2, no. 2 (1979): 183–94.

Solanas, Valerie. "SCUM (Society for Cutting Up Men) Manifesto." In *Radical Feminism: A Documentary Reader,* edited by Barbara Crow, 201–22. New York: New York University Press, 1967/2000.

Spampinato, Erin. "The Literary Roots of the Incel Movement." *Electric Lit,* May 24, 2018. https://electricliterature.com/the-literary-roots-of-the-incel-movement-4ba183b9c9c5.

Spillers, Hortense. "Interstices: A Small Drama of Words." In *Pleasure and Danger: Exploring Female Sexuality,* edited by Carole S. Vance, 73–100. London: Routledge and Kegan Paul, 1984.

Springer, Kimberly. *Living for the Revolution: Black Feminist Organizations, 1968–1980.* Durham, NC: Duke University Press, 2005.

Stallings, L. H. *Funk the Erotic: Transaesthetics and Black Sexual Cultures.* Champaign: University of Illinois Press, 2015.

Steiner, A. L. *Puppies and Babies.* University of Southern California, 3001 Gallery, 2012.

Stewart, Kathleen. *Ordinary Affects.* Durham, NC: Duke University Press, 2007.

Stockton, Kathryn Bond. *The Queer Child, or, Growing Sideways in the Twentieth Century.* Durham, NC: Duke University Press, 2009.

Stoler, Ann Laura. *Race and the Education of Desire: Foucault's History of Sexuality and the Colonial Order of Things.* Durham, NC: Duke University Press, 1995.

Storms, Michael. "Sexual Orientation and Self-Perception." In *Advances in the Study of Communication and Affect, Vol. 5: Perception of Emotion in Self and Others,* edited by Patricia Pliner, Kirk R. Blankstein, and Irwin M. Spigel, 165–80. New York: Plenum Press, 1979.

———. "Theories of Sexual Orientation." *Journal of Personality and Social Psychology* 38, no. 5 (1980): 783–92.

Subramaniam, Banu. *Ghost Stories for Darwin: The Science of Variation and the Politics of Diversity.* Champaign: University of Illinois Press, 2014.

"Tammy Rae Carland: Lesbian Beds." *A Simple, Frugal Heart Blog.* 2011. http://thistlebirdhex. tumblr.com/post/13747149601/tammy-rae-carland-lesbian-beds-the-series-was.

Third World Women's Alliance. "Goals and Objectives." *Triple Jeopardy* (September–October 1971): 8.

Thorne, Barrie. "Re-Visioning Women and Social Change: Where Are the Children?" *Gender and Society* 1, no. 1 (1987): 85–109.

Tinsley, Omise'eke Natasha. *Thiefing Sugar: Eroticism between Women in Caribbean Literature.* Durham, NC: Duke University Press, 2010.

Torpy, Sally. "Native American Woman and Coerced Sterilization: On the Trail of Tears in the 1970s." *American Indian Culture and Research Journal* 24, no. 2 (2000): 1–22.

Traina, Cristina L. H. *Erotic Attunement: Parenthood and the Ethics of Sensuality between Unequals.* Chicago: University of Chicago Press, 2011.

Tronto, Joan C. "Age-Segregated Housing as a Moral Problem: An Exercise in Rethinking Ethics." In *Mother Time: Women, Aging, Ethics,* edited by Margaret Urban Walker, 261–77. New York: Rowman and Littlefield, 2000.

Tuck, Eve, and K. Wayne Yang. "Decolonization Is Not a Metaphor." *Decolonization: Indigeneity, Education & Society* 1, no. 1 (2012): 1–40.

Tucker, Angela. *(A)sexual.* New York City: Big Mouth Films, Arts Engine, 2011.

Ussher, Jane M. *Managing the Monstrous Feminine: Regulating the Reproductive Body.* London: Routledge, 2006.

Valk, Anne M. "Living a Feminist Lifestyle: The Intersection of Theory and Action in a Lesbian Feminist Collective." *Feminist Studies* 28, no. 2 (2002): 303–32.

Van Houdenhove, Ellen, Luk Gijs, Guy T'Sjoen, and Paul Enzlin. "Asexuality: Few Facts, Many Questions." *Journal of Sex & Marital Therapy* 40 (2014): 175–92.

Vicinus, Martha. *Intimate Friends: Women Who Loved Women, 1778–1928.* Chicago: University of Chicago Press, 2004.

*The View* (talk show). New York City: ABC, January 15, 2006.

Wallace, Lee. *Lesbianism, Cinema, Space: The Sexual Life of Apartments.* New York: Routledge, 2009.

Warner, Michael. *Publics and Counterpublics.* Cambridge, MA: MIT Press, 2002.

———. *The Trouble with Normal: Sex, Politics, and the Ethics of Queer Life.* Cambridge, MA: Harvard University Press, 1999.

Waterman, Emily. "Reactions of College Students to the Sexuality of Older People." *Journal of Student Research* 1, no. 1 (2012): 46–50.

Watters, Yulia, and Tommie V. Boyd. "Sexuality in Later Life: Opportunity for Reflections for Healthcare Providers." *Sexual and Relationship Therapy* 24, no. 3–4 (2009): 307–15.

Weisskopf, Susan (Contratto). "Maternal Sexuality and Asexual Motherhood." *Signs: Journal of Women in Culture and Society* 5, no. 4 (1980): 766–82.

Wendell, Susan. "Old Women Out of Control: Some Thoughts on Aging, Ethics, and Psychosomatic Medicine." In *Mother Time: Women, Aging, Ethics,* edited by Margaret Urban Walker, 133–50. New York: Rowman and Littlefield, 2000.

———. *The Rejected Body: Feminist Philosophical Reflections on Disability.* New York: Routledge, 1996.

Wilkins, James. "More Than Capacity: Alternatives for Sexual Decision Making for Individuals with Dementia." *The Gerontologist* 55, no. 5 (2015): 716–23.

Wilkinson, Eleanor. "The Romantic Imaginary: Compulsory Coupledom and Single Existence." In *Sexualities: Past Reflections, Future Directions,* edited by Sallys Hines and Yvette Taylor, 130–45. London: Palgrave Macmillan, 2012.

Willey, Angela. *Undoing Monogamy: The Politics of Science and the Possibilities of Biology.* Durham, NC: Duke University Press, 2016.

Williams, Cristan. "Radical Inclusion: Recounting the Trans Inclusive History of Radical Feminism." *TSQ: Transgender Studies Quarterly* 3, no. 1–2 (2016): 254–58.

Winnicott, Donald. *The Family and Individual Development.* London: Tavistock Publications, 1965.

Women's Commune. "Mind Bogglers." *Off Our Backs* 1, no. 9/10 (1970): 13.

Wong, Day. "Asexuality in China's Sexual Revolution: Asexual Marriage as Coping Strategy." *Sexualities* 18, no. 1–2 (2015): 100–116.

Young Lords Party. *Palante* 2, no. 10 (1970).

———. *Palante* 2, no. 15 (1970).

———. "Thirteen Point Program and Platform / Programa de 13 Puntos y Platforma." *Palante* 2, no. 2 (1970): 18–19.

———. "Young Lords Party Position Paper on Women." *Palante* 2, no 12 (1970): 11–14.

Yule, Morag A., Lori A. Brotto, and Boris B. Gorzalka. "A Validated Measure of No Sexual Attraction: The Asexuality Identification Scale." *Psychological Assessment* 27, no. 1 (2015): 148–60.

# INDEX

discrimination, 4, 8–10, 9 fig. o.2, 38, 85;
as fatigue, 101–2; and feminisms, 33–62;
feminist and queer approaches, 14–19;
growing into asexuality, 31, 97, 102–3, 110;
and lesbianism, 63–88; online, 4, 19; and
pathologization, 11–12, 14, 57, 64, 68, 86;
percentage of population, 13, 146n51; in
the plural, 11, 14, 39; politics and identity,
37–38; and pride parades, 4, 10; racism
within the community, 10; as resistance, 16–17, 33–62; as valid, 2; as wasted
whiteness, 19. *See also* erotics; political
asexuality/celibacy

asexuality-as-ideal, 16, 41, 94, 104, 140

"Asexuality Identification Scale" (Brotto), 13,
146n53

Ashley X, 95

Atkinson, Ti-Grace, 36, 40, 52, 53–55, 150n13

attraction, 3, 4, 27; aesthetic attraction, 5;
aromantic attraction, 4–5; asexual attraction, 135–36; attraction model of sexual
identity, 4–6, 27; and *DSM*, 14; and *Frances Ha* (film), 131–32, 135–36; and gender,
5, 6; and Kinsey, 12; romantic attraction,
4–5; sensual attraction, 5; sexual attraction, 4, 5, 13, 19, 26, 27; subjective attraction, 13

autism, 15

Awkward-Rich, Cameron, 1–2, 24, 28

Bambara, Toni Cade, 17, 30, 35, 41, 42, 45–47,
49, 50, 54, 138

Barounis, Cynthia, 74, 92

Barthes, Roland, 99

Bartky, Sandra Lee, 126–27

BDSM, 11, 105, 106

Bear, Tracy, 24, 25

Beauvoir, Simone de, 55

Bechdel, Alison, 68

bed, the, 31, 33, 34 fig. 1.1, 58, 62, 68, 70 fig.
2.1, 70 fig. 2.2, 77–84, 79 fig. 2.3, 81 fig.
2.4, 88, 119, 126, 127, 132. *See also* lesbian
bed death

bedroom, the, 23, 34 fig. 1.1, 59, 80, 81 fig.
2.4, 82–84. See also *Lesbian Bedrooms II*
(Lasky)

Bell, Shannon, 126

Bennett, Bob, 47

Berlant, Lauren, 16, 31, 64, 71, 86–87, 135; and
cruel optimism, 71; and the good life,
71, 135; and sex without optimism (with
Edelman), 31, 64, 86–87

Bersani, Leo, 72, 97

Berson, Ginny, 59

*Big Bang Theory, The* (tv show), 15

biopolitics, 21, 67, 71–72, 110, 114; and Agamben, 116; chronobiopolitics, 114; and
desexualization, 67, 71, 114, 116, 123–24;
and disgust, 118; and disposability, 114,
116; and Foucault, 115; and sexuality, 21,
110, 114, 115

biopower, 21, 115

birth control, 35, 40, 41, 80, 83

bisexuality, 5, 6, 8, 12, 24, 29

black feminisms, 22, 42–43, 47, 53–54, 55, 75

Black Power, 35, 39, 42, 44, 47, 52, 53, 54, 55

*Black Woman, The* (Bambara), 41, 42, 44,
45, 54

Bogaert, Anthony, 12–13, 14, 145n47

*BoJack Horseman* (tv show), 15

Bolick, Kate, 29, 128

Boston marriages, 29, 30, 65, 75–76, 136

Bradway, Katherine, 123

Brake, Elizabeth, 5, 47

Breines, Winifred, 41–42

Brotto, Lori, 13, 146n52, 146n53

*Brown and Gray* (jnramos), 10

Brown, Cole, 4

Brown, Helen Gurley, 40

Brown, Rita Mae, 58–59

Bunch, Charlotte, 59

Carland, Tammy Rae, 31, 65, 78–80, 79 fig.
2.3, 82–84, 88, 157n54

Carrigan, Mark, 10

Carter, Julian, 19

Castle, Terry, 75

celibacy, 29, 130; and black history, 43–45;
clerical celibacy, 45, 104; imposed celibacy, 44; incel, 32, 137–41; tyrannical
celibacy, 32, 137–41; and whiteness, 43,
104. *See also* asexuality-as-ideal; political
asexuality/celibacy

68, 75, 76, 82, 84, 88, 90, 103, 110, 131, 135–36; beyond sexuality, 24; conflation with sexuality, 22–23; contra-Freud, 20–22; erotics of excess, 31–32, 112–15, 127, 129–32, 134–36; erotics of failure, 31, 63–65, 84–88; erotics of revolution, 30, 33–37, 43, 60, 62; Freudian, 3; and gender binary, 22–23; and Huffer, 21; and Indigenous erotics, 24, 25; intergenerational erotics, 31, 90–91, 99–103, 103–10; lesbian erotics, 58–62, 63, 75, 80, 82–84, 114; limits of, 26; Lordean, 3, 21–24, 25, 26, 27, 33–34, 47, 50, 54, 61, 62, 75, 140; and the mundane, 23–24; Platonian, 3, 20; and Sandford, 21; the superficially erotic, 22

Ettinger, Bracha, x, 109

Faderman, Lillian, 76

Fahs, Breanne, 16, 37–38, 101–2

failure, 30–31, 63–65, 68, 71, 73–74, 77, 84–88, 136

Fanon, Frantz, 134

Father Divine, 45

Feinberg, Leslie, 76

female sexual interest/arousal disorder (FSIAD), 11, 13, 14

Feminists, The (organization), 30, 36, 53–56, 58–59, 61, 138

Fields, Jessica, 90, 94

first wave feminisms, 29, 35

Flibanserin/Addyi, 13, 124

*Fosters, The* (tv show), 30, 65, 68–74, 70 fig. 2.1, 70 fig. 2.2, 88

Foucault, Michel, 21, 24, 29, 57, 114, 115–16

Fraiman, Susan, 100

*Frances Ha* (film), 31–32, 115, 131–36, 133 fig. 4.1

Freeman, Elizabeth, 110

Freud, Sigmund, 3, 20–22, 23, 93, 95, 100

Friedan, Betty, 52

friendships, 20, 22, 69, 75, 80, 127, 131; being friend-focused, 5; intimate friendships, 30, 65, 75–76, 131–36

frigidity, 11, 20, 29, 40, 57

Froide, Amy, 128

Furies, The (organization), 30, 36, 59, 138

Gallop, Jane, 100

gay men, 12, 16, 19, 72, 92, 158n7

gayness, 8, 11–12, 16, 19, 24, 29, 45, 65, 69, 72, 78, 86, 90, 92–93; and The Young Lords Party, 49

gender binary, 6, 22–23, 37, 45–46, 50–51, 53–54, 67, 80

Gerhard, Jane, 40

Gilmore, Ruth Wilson, 117

Goffman, Erving, 119

González-Torres, Félix, 77, 78

Gottschalk, Donna, 33, 34 fig. 1.1

gray asexuality, 6, 10, 27

group "X" (Kinsey), 12

Gupta, Kristina, 15, 66–67, 73, 146n62

Halberstam, Jack, 73, 87

"Haven for the Human Amoeba, The" (Yahoo! Group), 4

Hawkins Owen, Ianna, 16, 19, 41, 43–44, 94, 104, 117

Hefner, Hugh, 40

Hesford, Victoria, 39

heteronormativity, 16, 30, 37, 39, 43, 67, 69, 80, 86, 87, 102, 104, 108, 127, 129, 132, 134–35, 139

heteroromantic, 6

heterosexuality, 6, 11, 12, 15, 16, 17–19, 27, 32, 35, 39, 40, 53, 54, 55, 57, 58, 59, 60–61, 63, 66, 67, 75, 93, 98, 115, 122, 124, 127–30, 138; heterosexual presumption, 26, 120. See *also* compulsory heterosexuality

Hills, Rachel, 29

Hinderliter, Andrew, 13

HIV/AIDS, 72, 78, 92, 158n7

Holland, Sharon Patricia, 24

Holmes, Sherlock (character), 15

homonormativity, 69, 74, 86–87, 105, 106

homoromantic, 6

Hopkins, Pauline, 43–44

*House* (TV show), 17–19, 18 fig 0.3A, 18 fig 0.3B

Huffer, Lynne, 21

Huggins, Ericka, 44, 151n48

# ABNORMATIVITIES: QUEER/GENDER/EMBODIMENT

## SCOTT HERRING, SERIES EDITOR

This series explores the embodiment of gender identity and queerness within national and global frameworks of deviance that challenge hetero- and homonormative constructions of the body. The scope of the series is global and transnational, its time frame broad, and its focus interdisciplinary—from literary and cultural studies to history and anthropology and beyond.

* 9 7 8 0 8 1 4 2 5 5 4 2 1 *